THE WHOLE
9 MONTHS

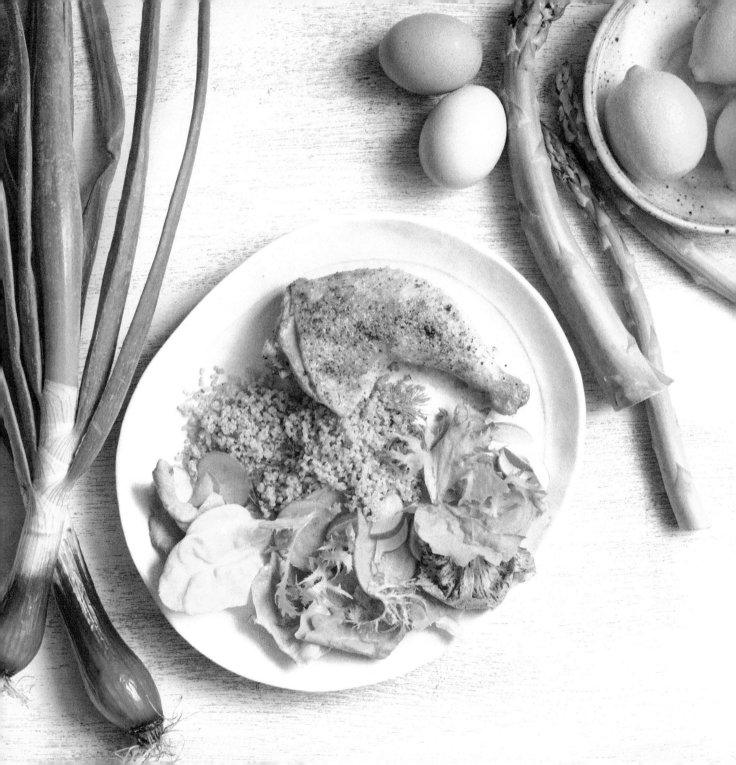

THE WHOLE

9

MONTHS

A Week-by-Week
Pregnancy Nutrition Guide with
Recipes for a Healthy Start

Jennifer Lang, MD

with recipes by Dana Angelo White, MS, RD, ATC

foreword by
Jessica Alba

SONOMA
PRESS

For general information on our other products and services or to obtain technical support, please contact our Customer Care Department within the United States at (866) 744-2665, or outside the United States at (510) 253-0500.

Sonoma Press publishes its books in a variety of electronic and print formats. Some content that appears in print may not be available in electronic books, and vice versa.

ISBN: Print 978-1-943451-48-7 | eBook 978-1-943451-49-4

To Sheila, Nico, and Sofia

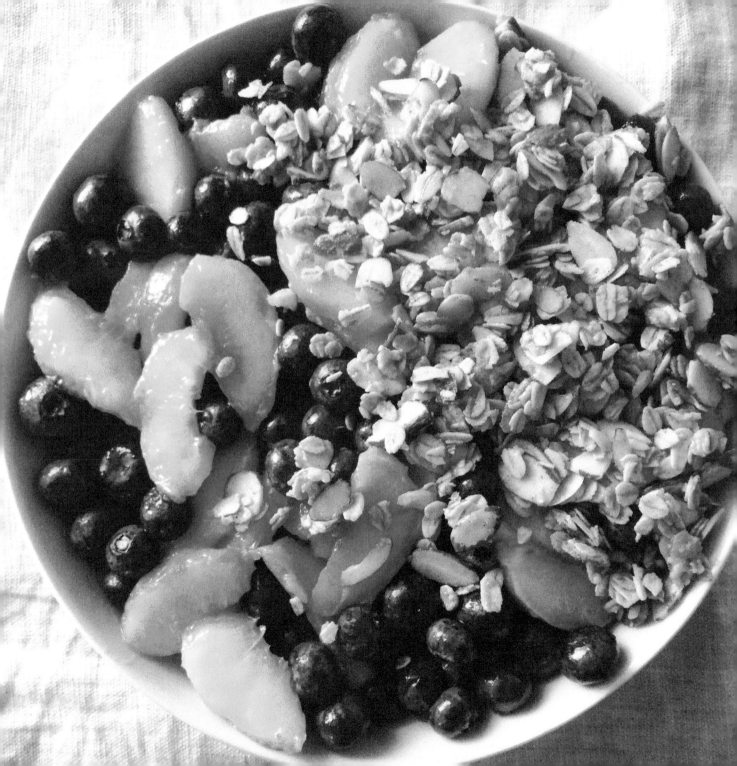

Contents

Foreword

I love everything about being a mom. Before having kids, I didn't realize it was possible to have this much love, joy, and happiness in my life. It's overflowing, unconditional, and selfless—and the most profound experience I've ever had.

But I didn't start out feeling that way when I was pregnant with my first baby, Honor. Honestly, it was a little scary and overwhelming. There's this tiny person inside of you that's completely dependent on you. Then, my motherly instincts kicked in (even before I had given birth) and I made it my mission to do everything possible to make sure my family had a healthy and safe environment.

This quest extended to helping all moms do what's best for their babies; in fact it drove me to start the Honest Company. I thought about the toxic chemicals that may contribute to conditions like asthma, allergies, autism, ADHD, and cancer, many of which are present in products that touch your baby (think diapers, cleaning products, even toys!). It became my life's mission to educate people about these hidden toxins and to offer safe alternatives.

Dr. Jennifer Lang and I have very similar health rules for moms: Know exactly what's going into and on your body. Creating a safe environment for your baby begins the day your baby begins to grow in the womb. As you'll learn in *The Whole 9 Months*, the food choices you make can have lasting effects on the long-term health of your children, including their brain and organ development, and even their future food preferences. Plus, how you eat during pregnancy can lay the foundation for good eating habits for life. Just think: if you develop their penchant for veggies early on, you probably won't have to

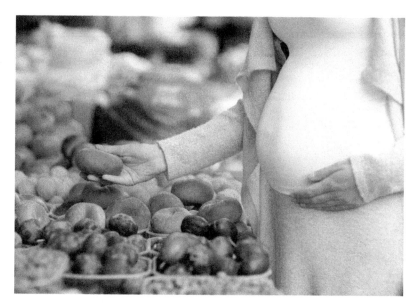

Creating a safe environment for your baby begins the day your baby begins to grow in the womb.

create a kids' meal *and* an adult meal—you will all be eating the same thing!

It can be daunting to sift through the claims on food packaging and to try to figure out what will nourish your family and what's just a gimmick developed to make you believe that a processed, additive-laden food is a smart choice. That's where this book comes in. Dr. Lang focuses on what you can and should eat—she's done all the hard work of research and makes choosing healthy food for yourself and your baby so very easy. It's the book I wish I'd had with my pregnancies with Honor and Haven.

As moms and health activists, Dr. Lang and I are crusaders for healthy eating and safer non-toxic home products. We both know the joys and anxieties of pregnancy firsthand, and I'm thrilled that Dr. Lang has put her valuable knowledge into these pages. This book provides fact-based advice that you can trust from a doctor who is also a mom. With this book in your hand, you are on your way to putting your health first and setting your baby up for lifelong wellness.

Jessica Alba

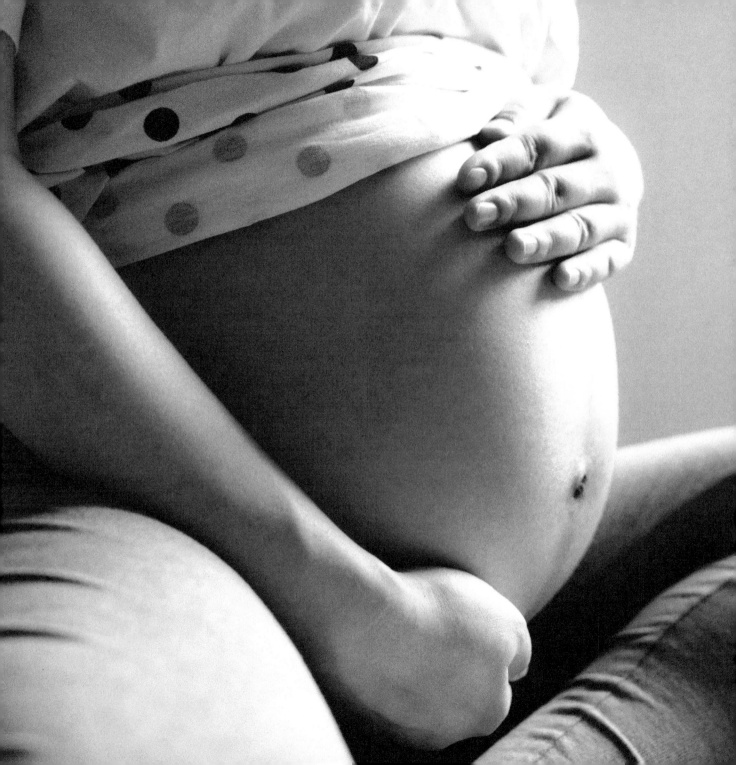

Introduction

Welcome to pregnancy, and to this book. Even though I've been through medical school, OB/GYN residency, gynecologic oncology (women's cancer surgery) fellowship, and counseled countless women on "eating healthy during pregnancy," I can honestly say I didn't have a true sense of what it all meant until I went through pregnancy myself.

This book is a guide that I hope will serve you as a vital tool and resource. My aim is to weave together science, real-life experience, and some truly delicious recipes that will nourish your baby and your body, setting both of you on a track for optimum healthy living, right from the start.

You may be familiar with the age-old debate regarding "nature versus nurture." Are we more influenced by heredity or our life experiences? In science-speak, this is sometimes referred to as "genes versus environment." The more scientists learn about the way environment influences our genes, the more clear it is that nurture can become nature, and vice versa. The two are inextricably linked.

How does this all affect me, you ask? Well, for example, science is showing us just how important eating well during pregnancy really is. It is probably the single most important thing we can control to set our body—and our baby's body—up for a healthy life. Through our eating habits during pregnancy, we can influence everything from our baby's chance of having a peaceful and healthy birth; to his taste palate in childhood and beyond; and even controlling, to some degree, his risk for developing diabetes or cardiovascular disease later in life.

Part of me is hesitant to call this a book about eating during pregnancy, because this is also a valuable guide for eating throughout life. Pregnancy happens to be a natural time when many women begin seriously considering what we are putting on, around, and inside our bodies. At this point, many of us become attuned to the idea of giving love, attention, and nourishment to our bodies for the first time, as we realize we are providing this love, attention, and nourishment to the developing baby inside us. I know this was a turning point for me!

But what exactly does that "love and attention" mean when we're talking about food? It's really very simple. Research shows that the key to healthy eating is a *whole foods, plant-based* approach. A provocative study published in the journal *Proceedings of the National Academy of Sciences* modeled how a plant-based diet is superior for the planet and for human health, capable of saving billions of lives, reducing global greenhouse emissions by 70 percent, and saving a trillion dollars in health care costs. If the majority of your diet is made up of foods that are minimally processed, come from the earth and mostly from plants, and you don't need a PhD in chemistry to decipher the ingredient list, you're already on the right track. And if not, you're still on the right track—you're here, aren't you? We'll walk through this journey together, and it'll be

a fun and eye-opening process that changes the way you think about food.

There's a bonus, too: Following a healthy balanced diet in pregnancy is going to have a transformational effect on *your* body as well. Everything that is good for your baby is good for you. Your thighs and tummy and boobs will be so grateful that they will reward you, because you won't have to try to drop excessive pregnancy weight or deal with more stretch marks. You will feel so much sexier if you have energy and can exercise—which you can do more readily when your legs aren't swollen and your back isn't sore. You will be kinder and more patient, as a partner and as a future mother, if your moods are not riding the roller coaster—tipped off by an over-indulgence in sugar or caffeine.

Another bonus to eating well is its trickle-down effect. When you reach the parenting phase of things, you will see that children model *everything*. If they see you choosing beautiful, colorful, fresh, and varied foods, they are much more likely to be comfortable making those same choices. Serving as an example with your healthy eating habits is one of the greatest gifts you can bestow on your baby, setting her up for success in so much that she does, even academically and athletically.

Food is powerful, and there are so many choices of products, brands, and cooking styles, but it is also something that we do not need to fret over. Even if you've never paid much

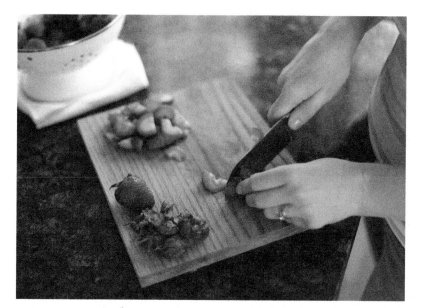

Food is powerful, and there are so many choices of products, brands, and cooking styles, but it is also something that we do not need to fret over.

attention to what you put in your body, this book is designed to make you feel more confident that you're making positive food choices, step-by-step, through your 40 weeks or so of pregnancy. I'm excited to share intriguing facts and foods to help empower you and your baby to thrive during this special time and beyond.

You are a pregnant woman in the twenty-first century; by definition, this means you undoubtedly have *a lot* going on in your life. Let's make healthy eating during pregnancy one less thing you have to worry about. After reading this book and making some simple shifts in your thinking and eating habits, I hope you'll become sufficiently inspired by your own good health and that of your baby that you'll keep these habits rolling for a lifetime!

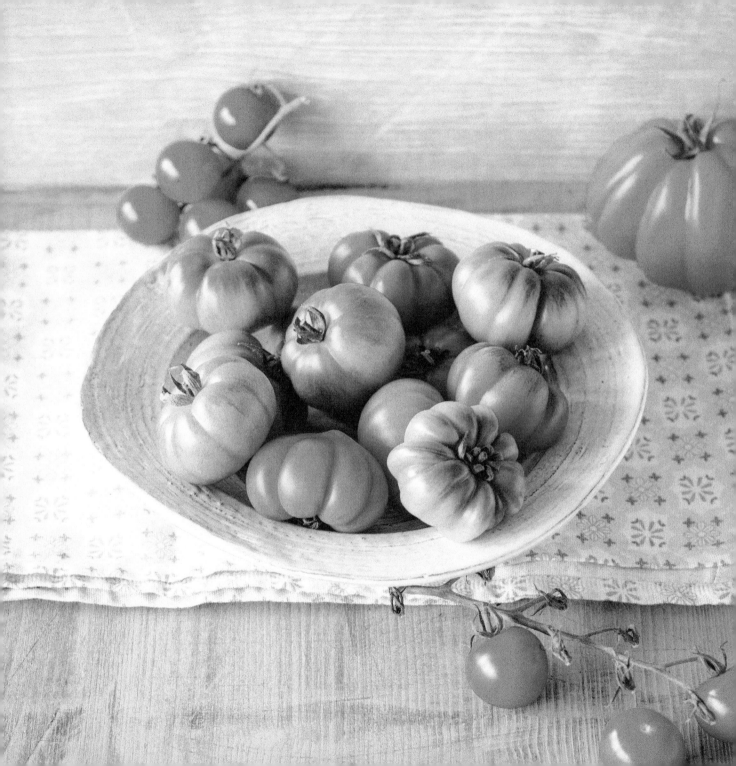

Part One

EATING DURING PREGNANCY

Yes, it's true. You are what you eat. And by intimate association, your baby is what you eat. You open your mouth and ingest food, and the nutrients in that food combine with stored nutrients to serve as the building blocks for your developing baby. This relationship sounds like a lot of pressure, but don't worry. Even if your diet up to this point has been less than optimum, you now have the perfect opportunity (and motivation) to completely re-create your internal environment for lasting benefits. Whether you've been eating well all along, or pregnancy is your inspiration for eating right, there is no more rewarding time than now to focus on the joys of good food.

one

HEALTHY BABY, HAPPY MAMA

If the majority of your diet comes from take-out, frozen dinners, prepared flavored rice in bright plastic bags, and mac and powdered cheese, you are not alone. This is exactly what dining has become for millions of Americans. But now you are eating for two and thinking about what's best for your baby, so let's talk about what foods will give you both everything you need to flourish.

GROWING A HEALTHY BABY

I was a second-year surgical fellow in gynecologic oncology, working insane hours, barely
sleeping, and just beginning to show my pregnancy bump under my scrubs, when I passed
a vending machine in the hospital. I saw the
image of a Diet Coke and it looked really good
to me. I approached the machine and dug into
the pocket of my lab coat for coins. Then it hit
me: the image of a little baby with a cord con-
necting that bottle of Diet Coke to its tummy.
If I drank this, I would literally be mainlining a
brown, fizzy, chemical soup into my little bean.
Nope, I said. *Walk away.*

Growing a healthy baby takes work. A lot of
that work is going on inside you as you go about
your business. Imagine every single chemical
reaction that takes place as your developing baby
grows from a sperm and egg to the single-cell
zygote, to the two-cell daughter blastomeres,
to the more complex embryo that now implants
itself in the wall of your uterus. What a miracle,
and we haven't even talked about fingers and
toes yet! Every single reaction at every stage
along this growth trajectory requires carbohydrates, fats, proteins, vitamins, minerals, water,
and oxygen. All of these get there because of you.
It's a huge responsibility, but it's also one of the
most empowering and extraordinary aspects of
human existence. With the right information

in your toolbox, you will meet this challenge
magnificently.

Brain Development

The brain is arguably the most essential organ
in determining who and how your baby will be
in this world. The developing brain is a virtual
sponge for essential nutrients, particularly
proteins, certain fats, zinc, copper, iron, iodine,
selenium, choline, vitamin A, and folate. Don't
worry about memorizing these—we'll talk
about good brain foods that contain these key
nutrients.

While early fetal brain development is very
"plastic" (able to correct itself after missing
nutrients are supplied), brain development in the
third trimester is very much dependent on the
present availability of key nutrient components.
Overall brain function, speed of processing,
motor function, and memory are just a few of the
brain-driven tasks that can be affected by nutrition. Long-lasting benefits can be seen if healthy
nutrition is a priority, particularly during Weeks
24 to 42 and the early neonatal period.

Clearly, we know more now about what's
good for baby than ever before. And admittedly,
all this information can seem overwhelming. But
the most important point is a simple one: Eating
a broad, varied diet based primarily on plants
and whole foods is the best way to ensure your
baby's brain has everything it needs to set itself
up for the academic decathlon. Also, getting good

prenatal care and soaking up information, like in this book, show you want to do the best for your baby—and that's a recipe for success!

Birth Weight

How much a baby weighs at birth is a result of a complicated blend of factors. Genetics and gestational age are just two of these factors. That saying "The more weight the mom gains during pregnancy, the more weight the baby will gain" is a myth. In fact, as adult obesity rates have increased, mean neonatal birth weights have actually started to decrease. Clearly many things are at play.

What is known for sure is that the birth weight of a child can be in part representative of the *quality* of nutrition provided during pregnancy. A healthy weight is associated with a healthy baby. And this is best achieved by doing our best to eat well during pregnancy, and providing the right nourishment for our baby to grow to the healthy weight her genetics intended.

Internal Systems and Organ Development

Certain nutrients are needed at different points along a baby's development so he can grow the internal organ systems he needs. Having all the building blocks available to the baby means that these organs will have what they need to form properly and function at their highest potential, and it also means that your body will be less depleted in the process. The baby's skeleton is a perfect example of this. If you are not consuming enough calcium in your diet, your baby will pull the calcium it needs for its own bones straight out of yours. While it's reassuring that our maternal bodies are already conditioned to "put baby first," optimally there should be enough nutrients in storage for both of you.

Long-Term Health

As a mother, you are your baby's first teacher. We teach our babies so much, including what to expect in the outside world. And this teaching starts earlier than birth! For example, if nutrients circulating through the placenta are in short supply, the baby is being set up metabolically to save and store nutrients when he is out in the world. We know now that babies who are either starved for nutrition or flooded with empty sugar-calories inside the womb are actually more likely to experience adult health problems such as cardiovascular disease and Type 2 diabetes. Both of these extremes are forms of malnutrition, and their effects can be long lasting. But the converse is also true: the effects of a nutritious foundation are long lasting and beneficial.

Personality

Will my baby be easygoing, or is she going to give us a run for our money? Will he have a competitive spirit or march entirely to his own drummer? There is no evidence that if you eat a certain way, your baby will show a certain personality type. At the same time, it's pretty clear that food can have a big effect on our own expressions of mood and personality. You may be familiar with the "crash" after a sugar high or the sluggishness sometimes you can feel after a big carb-filled meal. Scientists have discovered that the bacteria lining our gastrointestinal (GI) tract secrete neurotransmitters that affect how happy we feel. Generally, if you eat well, you will feel better and more emotionally stable, and even get better quality sleep. In doing so, you will help give your baby the same benefits.

Eating Habits

Starting in the second trimester, your baby is developing taste buds and a sense of smell. Already she is learning about flavors! The food choices you make directly affect what the baby is exposed to as she constantly sips and swallows the amniotic fluid that surrounds her. If you expose your baby to different tastes and spices, your baby will become more familiar with these things, and will therefore be more likely to accept them as an infant, child, and adult. You literally have the power to shape your baby's taste palate. But watch out: if sugary, salty, and savory are your go-to flavors, don't be surprised when that's all your four-year-old wants to eat!

GOOD FOR BABY, GOOD FOR YOU

It goes without saying that what is good for baby is good for you. But for some of us, there can be a disconnect between what we know to be good nutrition and what we actually consume. This begs the question, Why? I believe the answer lies in food addictions, fueled by poor-quality processed foods high in sugar, fat, and salt. If you follow a whole foods, plant-based diet, you will avoid addictive food traps and be able to easily maintain a healthy body weight.

I am not telling you to sacrifice for your baby. Quite the contrary. I want to inspire you with the idea that giving your body what it needs to thrive has countless rewards, both inside and outside of pregnancy.

Minimize Side Effects

Empty carbs and sodium-filled foods might give you the brief sensation of comfort, but if you really dial into how they make you feel just minutes after they go down, you may notice that they actually make you feel pretty crappy. Every time you eat simple sugars with a high glycemic index, you'll get a spike in energy that quickly leads to a crash. Sugar, and also caffeine, affect sleep habits and worsen the feeling of pregnancy-related fatigue. Sugars and salty foods make you retain excess water, leading to those swollen legs and feet that make you feel like you are dragging around lead pipes—which is hardly motivating when it comes time to do something fun and uplifting, like go for a hike in the sunshine or dance to your favorite music. You get the picture. If your diet is clean and nourishing, you will feel better and have the greatest potential of soaring through pregnancy.

Reduce Risk of Complications

If you maintain your ideal body weight and do not gain more weight than recommended during pregnancy, you will increase your chance of having a complication-free pregnancy and delivery. You will also reduce your risk of gestational diabetes, gestational hypertension, preeclampsia, and other conditions. But you don't have to deprive yourself. With the right ingredients—ones that satisfy and nourish—you can eat better than you've ever eaten before, and in fact, enjoy food more than ever. It's more about learning what foods pack the best nutritional punch, combining ingredients to create savory plates that you'll want to keep enjoying long after pregnancy, and building health-supportive habits that will stick with you and your baby.

Optimize Labor and Delivery

If you eat well in pregnancy and don't gain too much weight, you will be more likely to have a normal vaginal delivery. This is especially important if you are thinking about having another child in the future. Medical professionals are learning more and more about the benefits of vaginal delivery for both mother and baby.

If you stay mobile and within normal weight ranges, you will be able to move around more easily during labor and delivery, assume positions that allow the baby to move down the birth canal more freely, and minimize chances of delivery complications.

Finally, if you do need a C-section, doctors will be able to perform that surgery more quickly, efficiently, and safely for both you and your baby if your pregnancy weight is within the normal range.

Streamline Postpartum Recovery

If you can avoid having to recover from a major abdominal surgery while simultaneously dealing with all of the joys and challenges of new motherhood, that path is definitely the preferable one.

If you do have a C-section, and you followed a healthy diet during pregnancy, you are likely to see fewer complications like severe anemia, wound infections (and the need to take antibiotics), wound separation, and blood clots. A healthy diet puts you light-years ahead even with regard to your recovery.

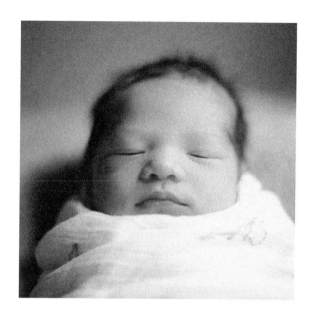

Maximize Long-Term Health

Don't let pregnancy be the thing that triggers a downward spiral into obesity and poor health. Conversely, if you can get on track with a healthy diet now, you will be in better shape to be a fit, active, and healthy mom who can take good care of your kids, and one day enjoy activities with your grandkids—sorry, that's probably rushing things!

For example, if you can support your baby's growing bones in vitro with healthy dietary sources of calcium so that calcium doesn't need to be pulled out of your body, you will be less likely to have weak bones later in life. A healthy diet now will provide you with lasting benefits.

DEALING WITH DISCOMFORT

I'm going to be a little unorthodox in this section. I hope my candor serves to make you feel better about things, especially if you are having a tough time getting in the food you think you need as you deal with nausea, constipation, or indigestion. If you don't feel like eating right now, it's okay. You definitely need to drink, but you actually don't need to eat that much, particularly in early pregnancy. Let's explore this.

Morning Sickness

Mother Nature is brilliant. Here is why it is in the best interest of our species to have some degree of nausea in the first trimester of pregnancy: *It is more important in the first trimester for you to avoid ingesting toxins than it is to take in nutrients for your baby's development.*

As long as you stay hydrated with sips of water, ginger tea, or even diluted coconut water (which has electrolytes and a small amount of naturally occurring sugar), your body will handle the rest. Try to swallow a simple prenatal vitamin once a day, 30 minutes after nibbling a whole-grain cracker (many pregnant women better tolerate the vitamin if taken at bedtime), and avoid exposure to drugs and alcohol, and with that, you are doing what you need to do. (See page 57 for antinausea tips.)

Constipation

Why do so many women get constipated during pregnancy? Well, the hormonal "soup" being pumped into your bloodstream from your placenta during pregnancy, along with aggressive iron supplementation found in certain prenatal vitamins (oh, yeah, and all those crackers), can definitely block you up and make you miserable.

Drink lots of water, and try squeezing a lemon into a big glass of water or hot tea every morning. This has benefits beyond relieving constipation (see box, page 23). Eat magnesium-rich foods, such as avocado, raw pepitas (shelled pumpkin seeds) or sunflower seeds, almonds, or black beans, or take a small magnesium supplement if you need to, and you will be surprised how your bowels thank you. Think of your entire diet as being a gentle cleanse for your intestines. If you are eating a whole foods, plant-based diet, you are, by definition, taking in lots of great stuff that help you maintain healthy bowel habits. Put the right things in, keep the wrong things out, and you probably won't have a problem with constipation.

Gassiness and Heartburn

When your plumbing isn't clogged, you will have an easier time with other common pregnancy complaints. High progesterone levels in pregnancy slow down bowel function, increase gastric emptying time, and relax the smooth muscle sphincters that generally keep things like stomach acid where they should be.

Gas is most bothersome to women when it causes those terrible sharp abdominal pains, but there's relief to be had. Most important, eating a fiber-rich diet that maintains a healthy gut microflora (the balance of bacteria in our GI tract) will make you much more comfortable with the gas issues. If you have an episode of uncomfortable gassiness, try switching to a non-carbonated liquid diet for a couple of days until everything starts moving again, then reintroduce soft, fiber-rich solids such as raspberries, apples, and oatmeal.

Papaya, pineapple, kiwi, and apples have beneficial digestive enzymes that are very helpful in preventing heartburn and are safe in pregnancy. You can also get help by focusing on alkaline foods like dark leafy greens, instead of acidic foods like meat, dairy, and processed sugars.

Did you know? Ginger can be your best friend for dealing with morning sickness. Just a few slices of peeled fresh ginger simmered in hot water for tea can provide relief from the most severe nausea and vomiting during pregnancy, with no adverse reactions.

Soften the Side Effects

You can alleviate those troublesome pregnancy maladies. Clever food choices, along with some other tricks, will go a long way in ensuring a comfortable nine-month journey.

FEEL THIS	TRY THIS
Fatigue	Take a nap, avoid foods with added sugar, and exercise moderately.
Swelling	Cut down on salty and sugary foods/liquids and bread products, drink lots of water with lemon, and exercise moderately.
Leg cramps	Take a warm bath with a cup of Epsom salts and a few drops of lavender essential oil before bedtime.
Hair changes	Up your intake of dark leafy greens and healthy plant fats (seeds, nuts, avocado). Prenatal vitamins also help.
Constipation	Drink a cup of hot water with squeezed lemon. Make yourself a fresh, organic green juice (see Dr. Jennifer's Green Smoothie, page 105).

CRAVINGS AND AVERSIONS

Have a craving for, or aversion to, a particular food? This is practically guaranteed at some point during your pregnancy. In fact, it's guaranteed in life. And pregnancy is life: it's a normal, natural state for a woman's body to be in. It does not require anything particularly different from what we require the rest of our nonpregnant time on this earth.

Everyone has cravings. Food companies count on this when they deliberately manipulate salt, sugar, and fat content to induce the craving phenomenon. If you crave potato chips, try not to eat a whole bag. If you crave Skittles while you are pregnant, try your best not to eat them. Think about each one of your cravings and how it will affect your baby. If it doesn't seem like a good idea to give a particular food to her, you probably shouldn't give it to yourself.

The wonderful news in all of this is that you can change what you crave. Like for any pattern of behavior, the longer you go without artificially flooding your taste buds with flavors that are not found anywhere in nature, the easier it will be not to seek these things out. Do listen to your body, though, and think creatively; that way, when you have a craving, you can offer it the

Drowning Out the Noise

You will discover when you're pregnant that everyone has an opinion. And somehow, well-meaning family, friends, and strangers have come to see your growing abdomen as a "welcome" sign for not only touching you, but also dispensing unsolicited advice. Unless the person is a friend who knows you very well and understands some of your personal issues, just nod and smile politely and move on, just like you will do when someone tries to tell you her scary, painful birth story.

Admittedly, it can be confusing and sometimes overwhelming to process all of the noise and advice out there. This book is medically sound advice written with love from someone who has "been through it," three times as a mother and many times as a doctor. When it comes to food, diets work when they are simple, clear, and intuitive. In this case, by "diet," I mean the food you eat to sustain yourself—not necessarily the foods you eat to lose weight. If you really tap into how you feel when you consume different foods and eat mindfully, your baby and your body will tell you what they need to thrive.

healthy version. (See page 66 for wholesome substitutes for your cravings.)

Aversions are less concerning than cravings. As long as you are not filling yourself with empty calories that are devoid of any nutrients, there are no foods that you absolutely *must* have. If you don't like it, don't eat it.

STAYING ACTIVE

Whether you are currently inactive or you follow a robust workout regimen, most physical activity during pregnancy is great for you and baby. Endorphins are "feel good" hormones that release during exercise; we can all use more of them, right? Baby benefits from these hormones as well. To boot, increased exercise is associated with lessened body aches and back pain, better sleep, and easier delivery, to name a few. Talk to your practitioner about your physical goals; he or she may have advice based on your history and special needs.

I know a brilliant psychotherapist with a large private practice in New York City who once told me that he will not even begin to work with a client unless the person commits to daily exercise. I am not exaggerating when I tell you that *everything gets better* when you move. So find your thing that feels like play and do it every day. It will begin a positive cascade that transforms your life.

Perceived Exertion Chart

Unless you are an elite athlete in training, don't worry about heart rate zones when you exercise. It is more meaningful to think big-picture about how you feel as you are engaging in an activity. In the sports-medicine world we call this the "Perceived Exertion Scale." When you are pregnant, you will want to keep your physical activity within the 2 to 8 range.

10   **Extremely Difficult Activity**
Maximal effort, out of breath, can only be sustained in short bursts

9   **Very Difficult Activity**
Breathing very hard, can talk only in short one-word answers, sweating profusely

7–8   **Difficult Activity**
Can speak a sentence or two at a time, but breathing hard and likely sweating

4–6   **Moderate Activity**
Breathing harder, but can still carry on a conversation

2–3   **Light Activity**
Easy breathing, feels like it could be done all day.

1   **No Activity**

two

HEALTHY EATING FOR TWO

In Chapter 1, we talked about the importance of eating healthy. Now let's explore the kinds of nutrients, and the foods they fill, that will maximize your energy levels, health, and baby's development at each stage of this extraordinary journey. In this chapter, the discussion primarily focuses on large-scale patterns of eating rather than breaking things down into individual nutrients.

THE WHOLE TRUTH

A "whole-foods diet" means that what you eat is mostly made up of real food that has been minimally processed. Think of whole foods as those foods that look exactly as nature intended. Fruits and vegetables. Whole grains. Eggs. Nuts and seeds. I feed my family a whole foods, plant-based diet because I believe this is truly the healthiest—and most delicious—way of eating. Small quantities of organically raised animal products can certainly be a part of a healthy plant-based diet, but they are by no means necessary. It is hard to argue with the science behind keeping plants as the primary source for our nutrition.

Whole foods either do not have an ingredient list (because they are not a package; they are a food), or when you read the ingredient list, you are reading a list of real foods, not chemical food additives. The "minimally processed" concept means that in their cooking, grinding up, and packaging, these foods do not lose a significant amount of their natural makeup. I also believe in taking at least 50 percent of your diet from "living foods"; that is, fresh and uncooked plants, which tend to have the highest vitamin, mineral, and phytonutrient content.

Unless you live in one of the communities in the United States referred to as a "food desert," where it is very hard to find fresh, real foods (in which case you could make your own garden or organize a community co-op garden), it is not difficult or expensive to eat healthy foods. Perhaps you've heard the advice to "shop the perimeter" of the grocery store. This is sound advice. It's where grocers keep the real foods that nourish and satisfy you, such as fresh fruits and vegetables, fresh dairy, and fresh meats. The center shelves of the store are filled with highly processed packaged items masquerading as food. Shopping the perimeter will not only keep you healthier; it will help you save money by avoiding the temptation of all those pricey, processed sugar-, salt-, and fat-filled foods that trigger you to buy more of them and thereby consume more calories.

Did you know? The Environmental Working Group has an online tool that rates more than 80,000 food products based on three broad criteria: nutritional value, ingredients, and processing concerns. Foods are rated from 1 (best) to 10 (worst), and you can even compare products by brand. This tool is a great way to learn the true value of foods, including fruits, vegetables, and even those veggie chips or a favorite packaged muffin mix, as well as discover whether there are more healthy options available. Visit ewg.org/foodscores.

A PLANT-BASED PREGNANCY

In 2013, a study in the *Permanente Journal* recommended a regimen consisting mostly of nutrient-dense plant foods—specifically known as a plant-based diet—because it leads to significant health benefits, including lower body weight and decreased cancer risk and heart disease. This diet maximizes consumption of foods from plants while minimizing or eliminating animal foods (including dairy and eggs) and processed foods like bleached flour, refined sugar, and processed oils. Essentially, it's a whole-foods diet with a plant focus.

While vegan and vegetarian diets fall under this category, a plant-based diet allows for flexibility since it leaves room for a small amount of animal product consumption. I've been vegetarian and vegan for most of my life, including through all three of my awesome pregnancies. My kids are thriving in every way and have never needed to take antibiotics. I find that eating a plant-based diet is one of the easiest ways to avoid excessive toxin exposure, including those that can lead to food-borne illnesses. And on a more positive note, plant-based eating is an aesthetically beautiful and delicious way to dine: it leaves you lean, filled with energy, and prospering in mind, body, and spirit.

If you cut out animal products, but then eat a highly processed diet with lots of food additives, preservatives, and sugars, you will be severely malnourished. But if you stick to a balanced whole-foods diet that comes from plants, it is quite difficult to be malnourished. There is more than enough protein found in nuts, seeds, legumes, and whole grains to meet our dietary needs. Plenty of calcium can be derived from plant foods like dark leafy greens, cruciferous vegetables, and fortified almond or soy milk. Vitamin B_{12} can be obtained from fermented foods like tempeh, miso, or nutritional yeast. If you find yourself nutritionally deficient in any way, try first to enhance your diet with plant-based food items, but if you need to, you can take a supplement or two to make up the difference.

Although some recipes in this book include animal products as ingredients, most can be easily converted to plant-based variations by substituting products like tofu for eggs and meat, or almond milk for cow's milk.

Did you know? The American Heart Association currently recommends no more than 25 grams of sugar per day for women. That is 6 teaspoons, or 100 calories worth. However, the average American consumes an average of 19 teaspoons of sugar per day.

BASIC PRINCIPLES FOR
Healthy Eating

You can keep it simple by eating an apple, or you can take 5, 10, even 20 whole-food ingredients and make a gourmet dish with complex flavors. You can go sweet or savory or spicy or creamy. You can love food more than ever. And you can *do it all* without processed foods. Here is a list of basic principles of healthy eating (in pregnancy and in life):

KEEP IT REAL Base your diet on fresh, whole, unprocessed foods that grow out of the earth.

EAT MINDFULLY Think about what you are putting in your body and why.

CHOOSE WISELY Seek out quality calories, and avoid empty ones.

EAT THE RAINBOW Eat many varieties and colors of fresh, living plants each day.

PACK THE PANTRY Keep your kitchen stocked with healthy foods.

BE PREPARED Keep easy, healthy snacks on hand to grab on the go.

DON'T BEAT YOURSELF UP An occasional food slip is forgivable.

LISTEN TO YOUR BODY Eat when you're hungry, and drink water when you're thirsty.

DON'T MICROMANAGE! There's no need to count calories, or to weigh or measure yourself.

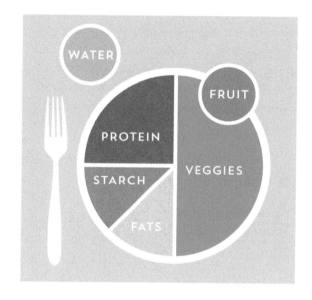

SUPPLEMENT YOUR DIET Take a good-quality prenatal vitamin containing DHA daily.

EAT MOSTLY VEGETABLES At least half of your plate should be filled with veggies.

READING FOOD LABELS

If you are reading a food label, it is usually because you are considering purchasing a packaged food product. It's hard to control what you're served in a restaurant or at an office lunch, but you can be the boss of what you bring into your home. If it isn't there to tempt you, you will reach for healthier choices, and over time, you will come to crave healthier choices.

Food labels are one big way that companies try to convince you a packaged product is healthy when really it is not. You can basically disregard any statement on the front label, with the exception of the USDA organic stamp. There are no standards or regulations for being able to call something "Natural" or "Healthy." Instead, turn over the product and read the back label.

First, look at the ingredient list. If it includes sugar in any form, it's better to pass. If you don't know what the ingredients are, again, take a pass.

Second, look at the "Nutrition Facts." How many servings are in one package? How likely is it that you won't eat the entire package? One devious trick used by food companies, to cut the amount of fat by 50 percent in a product, is to halve the suggested serving size. There you go, consumer. Voilà! 50 percent less fat!

Third, look at the details for fats, sodium, sugars, and protein, particularly the sodium (salt) and sugars. If a processed food is loaded with junk, you will see it in the sodium and sugar amounts. The American Heart Association recommends no more than 1500 milligrams of sodium per day for the average person and no more than 25 grams of sugar per day for women.

You will notice that sugar is one of the only items that has no "Percent of Daily Value" listed beside it. Food companies and industrial agriculture fought hard to keep this off labels, but this will soon change. The FDA announced new labeling guidelines that will go into effect by July 2018. The new design will highlight calories and servings, and will more realistically reflect the serving sizes that people actually consume. Added sugars will finally be declared as a percentage of daily value.

Nutrition Facts

8 servings per container

Serving size	2/3 cup (55g)

Amount per 2/3 cup

Calories 230

% DV*

12%	**Total Fat** 8g	
5%	Saturated Fat 1g	
	Trans Fat 0g	
0%	**Cholesterol** 0mg	
7%	**Sodium** 160mg	
12%	**Total Carbs** 37g	
14%	Dietary Fiber 4g	
	Sugars 1g	
	Added Sugars 0g	
	Protein 3g	

10%	Vitamin D 2mcg	
20%	Calcium 260mg	
45%	Iron 8mg	
5%	Potassium 235mg	

* Footnote on Daily Values (DV) and calories reference to be inserted here.

AN ORGANIC START

Consuming organic foods is important, especially when it comes to certain foods that are more affected than others by conventional farming methods. Look for the USDA organic label to differentiate organic products from ones that merely claim to be "natural," "healthy," etc. This is particularly important if you are consuming animal products, because animal fats bioaccumulate the chemicals, heavy metals, and toxins the animal has been exposed to. If you choose organic, by definition that means you are choosing products that are free from GMOs (genetically modified organisms), routine use of antibiotics and hormones, and harmful pesticides and fertilizers.

If you find it too expensive to buy organic all the time, then try to always choose organic for animal products, and purchase organic produce depending on the amount of pesticide residue. The most affected common produce are listed in the Environmental Working Group's Dirty Dozen (see list, page 33). These are considered the most important produce to buy organic. Conversely, if you want to know which conventionally grown foods have the lowest amounts of pesticide residue, refer to the Clean Fifteen (page 33). It is not as critical to buy organic Clean Fifteen foods.

With all the misinformation out there, it is important to educate ourselves on what is healthy and what is not. As you become increasingly conscious of the foods you eat and their sources, you may even find yourself inspired to become an activist in cleaning up our environment and food supply. What a great time to do so! With motherhood often comes a new sense of responsibility to our children and the planet we will pass on to them.

Organic Labeling

The USDA National Organic Program defines organic as that which is "produced by farmers who emphasize the use of renewable resources and the conservation of soil and water to enhance environmental quality for future generations. Organic meat, poultry, eggs, and dairy products come from animals that are given no antibiotics or growth hormones. Organic food is produced without using most conventional pesticides; fertilizers made with synthetic ingredients or sewage sludge; bioengineering; or ionizing radiation."

The USDA organic label means the farm where the product came from is adhering to a set standard of practices. Even so, only a small fraction of foods are ever tested for safety, which makes sourcing your foods locally from responsible sources quite important.

The statement "100% organic" means that every ingredient contained in the product is organic. "Organic" means that at least 95 percent of the ingredients are organic, and the remainder are GMO-free and not irradiated. "Made with organic ingredients" means at least 70 percent of the ingredients are organic, and the remainder are GMO-free and produced in compliance with strict guidelines.

Beyond Produce

Organic choices aren't just for fruits and vegetables. There are organic meats and dairy products and even organic herbs and oils. In fact, animal products—meats, dairy, eggs, and the like—are the most important part of your diet to only consume as USDA organic. Think about it this way: You can wash off some of the pesticides, hormones, or chemicals from the outside of the produce, but you can't wash it out of the inside of the animal product.

MEAT If you are going to choose only one thing in your diet to buy organically, make it your meat. Grass-fed and pasture-raised animals eat foods that nature intended them to eat. They are healthier and require fewer antibiotics. They also have a much lower *Escherichia coli (E. coli)* bacteria colony count, making them safer from a food poisoning perspective. Eating wild-caught fish avoids many of these issues. Conversely, factory-farmed meat and fish are bad for the animal, the earth, your body, and your baby.

DAIRY After meat, eggs and dairy are the second most important foods to consume organically for the same reasons as for meat. The feed given to animals makes it into the milk these animals produce and the eggs they lay. And here you can relate, since this concept works just like pregnancy—a mother's nutritional intake during pregnancy affects the health of the baby exactly the same way.

OILS While organic is the best way to purchase oils, it is not as critical as in the case of animal products. But there are other issues and benefits related to oils. Think of oils like fruit juices: they are best raw, minimally processed, and used in moderation. Different plant oils have different fat profiles. Some are higher in saturated fats (like coconut oil), polyunsaturated fats (sunflower oil), and monounsaturated fats (olive oil and sesame oil). Some are particularly rich in omega-3s (like flax oil), some have higher levels of vitamin E (like almond oil).

THE
Dirty Dozen and Clean Fifteen

The Environmental Working Group (EWG) is a nonprofit, nonpartisan organization dedicated to protecting human health and the environment. Its mission is to empower people to live healthier lives in a healthier environment. This organization publishes an annual list of the twelve kinds of produce, in sequence, that have the highest amount of pesticide residue—the Dirty Dozen—as well as a list of the fifteen kinds of produce that have the least amount of pesticide residue—the Clean Fifteen.

The Dirty Dozen

The 2016 Dirty Dozen includes the most important produce to buy organically:

1. Strawberries
2. Apples
3. Nectarines
4. Peaches
5. Celery
6. Grapes
7. Cherries
8. Spinach
9. Tomatoes
10. Bell peppers
11. Cherry tomatoes
12. Cucumbers
+ Kale/collard greens
+ Hot peppers

The Dirty Dozen list contains two additional items—kale/collard greens and hot peppers—because they tend to contain trace levels of highly hazardous pesticides.

The Clean Fifteen

The least critical to buy organically are the "Clean Fifteen" list. The following are on the 2016 list:

1. Avocados
2. Corn
3. Pineapples
4. Cabbage
5. Sweet Peas
6. Onions
7. Asparagus
8. Mangos
9. Papayas
10. Kiwi
11. Eggplant
12. Honeydew
13. Grapefruit
14. Cantaloupe
15. Cauliflower

PREGNANCY-SAFE
Eating

Pregnancy is an extraordinary phenomenon. Perhaps you feel like your body has been hijacked. Add to that the pregnancy hormonal roller-coaster ride, along with the life-changing promises, plans, and contemplations of new motherhood, and it can be quite overwhelming. There's a lot of information, advice, and hype circulating out there, and it's easy to get misled by the myths. Here are some general guidelines for what is safe and unsafe regarding foods:

	EAT		DON'T EAT
Fish/Seafood	Wild salmon, sardines, mussels, rainbow trout, max. 8 to 12 ounces, or 2 to 3 servings, per week		Albacore and bluefin tuna, king mackerel, swordfish, tilefish, shark, sushi
Meat	Organic grass-fed, free-range meats		Factory-farmed meat, raw meats, deli meats
Cheese	Organic pasteurized cheese		Unpasteurized cheese, processed cheese, factory-farmed cheese
Eggs	Well-cooked organic eggs with DHA/omega-3		Raw eggs, conventional (factory-farmed) eggs
Fruits/ Vegetables	Organic fruits and veggies, conventional fruits and veggies from the EWG Clean Fifteen list (page 33).		Nonorganic produce from the EWG Dirty Dozen list (page 33).

Oils to avoid completely include partially hydrogenated vegetable oils (containing cardiotoxic trans fats), and oils like canola, which are extensively processed. Also avoid oils made from GMO corn or soybeans and oils from animal products, since heavy metals, dioxins, and herbicide and pesticide residues get concentrated in animal fat.

CHECKING THE SCALE

It's not necessary or helpful to weigh yourself frequently and to obsessively focus on the number on the scale. If you started pregnancy either severely underweight or overweight/obese, you may want to step on the scale once a week throughout your pregnancy, just to make sure there are no big surprises. Your doctor or midwife will weigh you at each prenatal appointment, so if your weight gain goes off the anticipated track, this will be flagged. Most normal-weight women carrying singleton (single fetus) pregnancies should gain between 25 to 35 pounds over the course of their pregnancy. For women carrying twins, that range will be more like 35 to 55 pounds.

See the following table for recommended weight gain according to pre-pregnancy Body Mass Index (BMI) from the Institute of Medicine (2009). BMI data are from the World Health Organization (WHO).

BMI (KG/M²)	TOTAL WEIGHT GAIN RANGE (LBS)	RATES OF WEIGHT GAIN*
PRE-PREGNANCY BMI : UNDERWEIGHT		
<18.5	28–40	1 (1–1.3)
PRE-PREGNANCY BMI: NORMAL WEIGHT		
18.5–24.9	25–35	1 (0.8–1)
PRE-PREGNANCY BMI: OVERWEIGHT		
25.0–29.9	15–25	0.6 (0.5–0.7)
PRE-PREGNANCY BMI: OBESE		
≥30.0	11–20	0.5 (0.4–0.6)

*2nd and 3rd trimester (mean range in lbs/wk)

In general, Americans are overly preoccupied with food and eating. We will not starve, nor will our babies, if we go a few hours between meals. However, if you have a job where your access to food or liquid is limited, it's wise to plan ahead and bring a little baggie of nuts or a piece of fresh fruit and a BPA-free water bottle with you. This will help you prevent your blood sugar from dropping, which could lead you to grab something unhealthy when you suddenly feel famished. Here's a myth worth dispelling: You do not need to "eat for two" during pregnancy. For a singleton pregnancy, 300 extra calories a day from the second trimester to full term are all you need.

KEY NUTRIENTS FOR A HEALTHY PREGNANCY

We use the word *nutrient* a lot, but what does that actually mean? The medical definition of nutrient is "a constituent of food necessary for normal physiologic function." There are six main classes of nutrients you need to consume: water, proteins, carbohydrates, fats, vitamins, and minerals.

Water

Yes, water is a nutrient, and it's an important one. Our adult bodies are composed of about 65 percent water. We need water for nearly every physiologic function. You can derive a good amount of water from your foods, particularly if you are eating fresh, raw fruits and vegetables. Otherwise, drink water in the form of pure filtered water stored in glass (with no added sugars or artificial sweeteners). Aim for the equivalent of about 12 eight-ounce glasses per day from all sources.

Carbohydrates

These macronutrients, often referred to as "carbs," are classified as either simple or complex, and should form the majority of what gives us energy in a healthy diet. This is especially true during pregnancy. Carbohydrates have always (even in Paleolithic times) formed the basis of almost every culture's diet. It is important to get enough healthy carbohydrates during your pregnancy to ensure the baby's good neurologic development and overall health. Fiber is a carbohydrate that actually goes through your digestive system undigested and does not contain calories but is equally essential. Let's explore the different types of carbs and which foods pack the best healthy carb punch.

SIMPLE CARBOHYDRATES are found in nature in things like fruits, where they are complemented and balanced by large amounts of water, fiber, vitamins, minerals, and phytonutrients. Since they are only made up of one or two sugar molecules (thus, their name "simple"), simple carbs are more rapidly broken down by the body and able to enter the bloodstream and utilized as a source of immediate energy. Milk contains the simple sugar, lactose. Raw honey, raw cane juice, and raw maple sap are examples of items that are very high in simple carbs and do not have much balance from fiber, fats, or proteins to modify the speed at which they are absorbed. These simple carbs should be taken in sparingly, but go ahead and eat a wide variety of fresh fruits and berries.

COMPLEX CARBOHYDRATES are made up of multiple sugar molecules linked together. These foods take the body a little longer to break down than simple carbs, and as such, provide a great source of sustained energy over time. Complex carbohydrates found in nature can be starchy, like rice, potatoes, oats, and other whole grains. Complex carbs can also be fibrous, like broccoli, asparagus, spinach, and mushrooms—these foods are also packed with a wide array of vitamins, minerals, prebiotics, and phytonutrients.

FIBER is a type of complex carbohydrate that is nondigestible. Edible fiber is found in unrefined whole plant foods, like fruits, vegetables, and whole grains. There is virtually no fiber in meat, dairy products, oils, or refined sugars.

PREBIOTICS are actually fibers that serve as food for **PROBIOTICS**, which are good bacteria that control harmful bacteria in the digestive tract. Naturally occurring prebiotics can be found in foods like bananas, garlic, onions, and asparagus. Some foods containing probiotics or that support probiotic growth include sauerkraut, kimchi, miso soup, coconut kefir, tempeh, and kombucha. A good probiotic supplement will also do the trick.

Did you know? Most adult women of reproductive age with normal physical activity levels have a recommended daily caloric intake of about 2,000 calories. You need zero extra calories in the first trimester, and only an average of 300 extra calories per day beginning in the second trimester through to full term for normal fetal growth and development.

Spa Water

Having trouble meeting your water quota? Ramp up the flavor and benefits from your water by adding the following foods—sliced, chopped, or whole—to a pretty glass pitcher full of water. You'll stay hydrated and help your body's immunity, skin, digestion, stress, bloating, and more:

- Berries of all kinds
- Cucumber
- Grapefruit
- Herbs like mint, rosemary, ginger, basil
- Lemon
- Lime
- Orange
- Pear
- Pineapple
- Pomegranate
- Strawberry

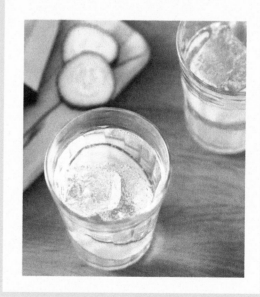

Fats

We are taught to fear fats, but fats are essential for human life. They make up the cellular membrane that surrounds and encloses every single cell in our bodies. They are required for the body's absorption of vitamins A, D, E, and K. So, fat itself is not bad. But some types of fats are healthier than others. Essential fatty acids (EFAs) cannot be created by the human body and need to be taken in through our diet. You may have heard of omega-3 and omega-6 fatty acids. These good and valuable fats are found in plants—particularly black beans and kidney beans, edamame, walnuts, flaxseed, chia seeds, and winter squash—as well as wild fatty fish, and are very important to our health. Other fats can be generated by the body, so they don't need to be ingested.

TRANS FATS exist in small amounts in animal fats like beef, lamb, and butterfat. It is not known how harmful naturally occurring trans fats may be. What *are* harmful to our bodies are the man-made trans fats that are produced when certain unsaturated vegetable oils are partially hydrogenated. This man-made process creates a substance that is not found in nature and should not be a part of our diets in any type or quantity.

SATURATED FATS are naturally occurring fats that are usually solid at room temperature. Meats and dairy products, as well as coconut oil and cocoa butter, have a high proportion of saturated fats. Though not as bad as trans fats, saturated fats are best kept to a minimum.

MONOUNSATURATED (OMEGA-9) FATTY ACIDS are not considered essential fatty acids because they can be produced by the body, but it is still beneficial to have omega-9 fatty acids in the diet. Good sources include nuts, avocados, and olive oil. They are protective against metabolic syndrome, cardiovascular disease, and stroke. Oils rich in monounsaturated fats can be an important source of the antioxidant vitamin E.

POLYUNSATURATED (OMEGA-3 AND OMEGA-6) FATTY ACIDS are needed by the body to synthesize other fats, including hormones. These are important to include in your diet, especially during pregnancy, and can be found in vegetable oils, nuts and seeds, fatty fish, and leafy vegetables.

Proteins

Proteins are built from amino acids, which are classified as either essential (need to be taken in through the diet) or nonessential (can be manufactured by the body). We need protein for every cellular function, and our baby needs a lot of protein to grow and develop optimally. But most Americans eat far too much protein. The average nonpregnant woman in the United States eats 70 grams of protein a day. This meets the Institute of Medicine's Dietary Reference

Index (DRI) for protein requirements in pregnancy. So, most women do not need to increase their protein consumption when they get pregnant. Good protein sources include nuts, seeds, legumes, whole grains, wild fish, and organic dairy products, eggs, and meats.

Vitamins

Vitamins are vital to our good health. Every vitamin has a specific role in the growth and function of our bodies. Synthetic and semi-synthetic vitamins have been mass produced and sold for decades, but their safety and value remain debatable. A whole-foods diet with lots of plant-based foods will provide you with plenty of vitamins. As an insurance policy in pregnancy, however, it is helpful to take a prenatal vitamin.

VITAMIN A   Vitamin A comes in two forms: retinol (found in animal products) and carotenoids (found in plants). Adequate vitamin A is essential for normal fetal internal organ development. But excess retinol can build up, causing toxicity. You can easily avoid this risk. Simply eat plenty of healthy carotenoid-containing vegetables. Think orange here: sweet potatoes, carrots, mangos, and cantaloupe are all good vitamin A foods, as are spinach, kale, iceberg lettuce, and red peppers. If you eat retinol-containing animal products, like meat and poultry, just do so in moderation. Avoid supplements containing retinol, as well as prescription drugs containing vitamin A or synthetic equivalents (like Accutane and Retin-A).

Eating for Twins (or More)

The biggest difference when you're carrying multiples is that your pregnancy-related symptoms may be magnified, and your caloric and nutritional needs somewhat amplified. Instead of growing one little being, you are growing two, or three, or sometimes more. You will also be seeing your obstetrician and/or perinatologist more frequently for prenatal care, so ideally, any weight concerns will be recognized and addressed appropriately. A good rule of thumb with multiples is to aim to gain at least 24 pounds by 24 weeks. If you hit this mark, you are very likely keeping up calorically with the needs of your developing babies. In the meantime, if you find that you are gaining either significantly less or more than an average of a pound per week, bring it to your doctor's attention.

VITAMIN B6 This good and kind vitamin is known to bring relief from the nausea and vomiting associated with morning sickness in the first trimester. It is also an important factor in metabolizing carbohydrates, fats, and proteins, and crucial to nervous system development. Foods rich in vitamin B6 include spinach, bananas, potatoes, chickpeas, and wild fish.

VITAMIN B9 (FOLATE/FOLIC ACID) Folate is a naturally occurring vitamin in foods such as dark leafy greens, whole grains, and beans. Folic acid is the synthetic crystalline version of this vitamin, which is contained in most prenatal vitamins and fortified foods. This important B vitamin is involved in DNA repair, cell division, and many other biological processes. It is also critical to the brain and spinal cord development of the fetus. Since we started fortifying our foods and recommending prenatal supplements with folic acid, rates of infant brain and spinal cord anomalies have decreased dramatically.

VITAMIN B12 This vitamin is helpful to the development of the brain and nervous system, and is closely related to folate. Adequate B12 levels ensure that folate can be metabolized and properly used by the body. Vitamin B12 is known to be protective against cleft lip and cleft palate, and is also essential to preventing maternal anemia. Some foods containing this vitamin include sauerkraut, kimchi, tempeh, spirulina, eggs, and milk.

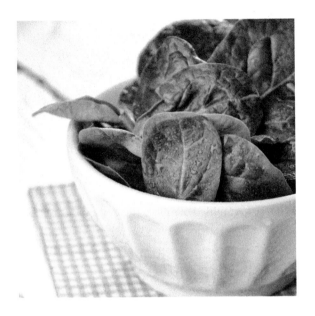

VITAMIN C Vitamin C is essential for creating collagen (the protein found in connective tissue), and is therefore important for normal fetal growth. It is involved in building healthy skin and connective tissues, and is an antioxidant with powerful immune capabilities. You may think of oranges in relation to vitamin C, but some perhaps more surprising foods providing vitamin C include strawberries, papaya, broccoli, Brussels sprouts, bell peppers, and guava.

Did you know? Much of the nutrition in root vegetables like potatoes and carrots is in the skin. Don't peel them—instead, scrub them well to retain maximum value.

VITAMIN D Vitamin D is manufactured in the skin by exposure to sunlight. This vitamin is needed for proper absorption and utilization of calcium and phosphorus in the body, and is essential for the growth of healthy bones and teeth. Recent recommendations to cover or use sunscreen on exposed skin may actually be contributing to low vitamin D levels. Especially during pregnancy, this vitamin is critical to both mom (prevents gestational diabetes) and baby (ensures skeletal development and full-term gestation). Sardines, chanterelle mushrooms, egg yolks, cheese, and of course sunlight are good sources of vitamin D.

CHOLINE Choline is not actually a vitamin. It is a vitamin-like micronutrient that is absolutely vital for numerous cell processes. Choline is particularly important during pregnancy to ensure proper development and functioning of the nervous system. It's also recommended early in pregnancy, along with folate and vitamin B$_{12}$, to prevent neural tube defects. Later in pregnancy, choline will enhance baby's brain development. Eggs, scallops, spinach, broccoli, and quinoa are among the many foods containing choline.

Did you know? Always wash fresh fruits and vegetables, regardless of whether they "have been washed," are "organic," or are "conventionally grown," to remove pesticides as well as dirt and germs that come from handling.

Minerals

Minerals are essential to every bodily function, from brain to heart to bowel. Their levels tend to be well regulated by the body, which is helpful as problems can arise with either a deficiency or an excess of most minerals. The kidneys do a lot of work maintaining this balance. Nurture good kidney health by drinking plenty of water and avoiding excess sugars and sodium.

It's also important to consider the quality of the soils in which our food is grown when we consider a food's mineral content. Conventional fertilizers and agricultural techniques degrade the soil mineral quality and contaminate groundwater supplies. Choose USDA organic as often as possible to maximize the nutritional value of your food.

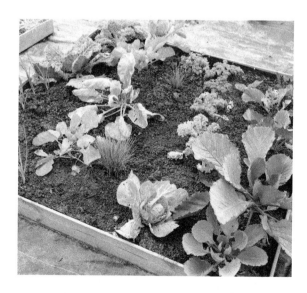

CALCIUM Calcium helps the baby grow a healthy skeleton and teeth, cardiovascular system, and heart rhythm. If you don't supply enough calcium in your diet, your growing baby will take the calcium it needs out of your bone stores, leaving you vulnerable. Conversely, getting adequate calcium during pregnancy actually protects your child from increased fracture risk later in life. Calcium is commonly associated with dairy products, but it can also be found in fortified almond or soy milk, broccoli, tofu, bok choy, and Chinese cabbage.

IRON Iron is required to make heme, the central component of hemoglobin, which is the part of the blood that carries oxygen around on your red blood cells. Iron is that vital. There has been, though, an overemphasis placed on iron in pregnancy. I encourage pregnant women to check their ferritin level (this reflects your iron stores), and take a supplement only if your level is low. Heme iron comes from animal sources and is more readily absorbed. Non-heme iron comes from both plants and animals. It is better absorbed (up to three times as well) by your body if you take it in along with a food or drink rich in vitamin C. Iron-rich foods include lentils, squash, and pepitas (shelled pumpkin seeds), black sesame seeds, dark leafy greens, and dried fruits, such as prunes and raisins.

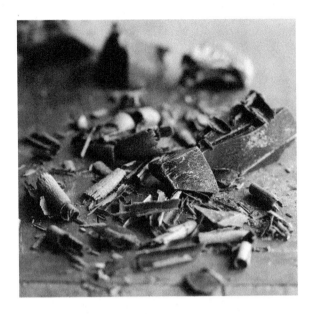

MAGNESIUM Magnesium is important for manufacturing the vitamin D absorbed via the body's exposure to sunlight. It's also beneficial for calcium absorption, normal bowel function, muscle relaxation, and mental calmness. Industrial agriculture (think fertilizers and pesticides, which empty the soil of micronutrients) and food processing, have led to a magnesium deficiency in our diets. To counter this, eat magnesium-rich plant foods, use occasional Epsom salts baths (to absorb magnesium sulfate through the skin), and consider taking a prenatal vitamin containing magnesium. Who can't benefit from a little additional muscle relaxation and mental calmness? You'll have a happier and healthier pregnancy for it. Magnesium is found in dark leafy greens (yes, you've seen a lot of these—part of what gives them their status as "superfoods"; see page 70), beans, nuts, seeds, fish, avocado, dried fruit, and dark chocolate, to name a few.

ZINC This mineral is essential for cell division, protein synthesis, nucleic acid metabolism (helps make DNA), and a healthy immune system. Unlike naturally occurring folate, folic acid can inhibit zinc absorption. For increased zinc absorption, try soaking nuts and legumes in filtered water before sprouting (see box on this page) or cooking them. In addition to nuts and legumes, some good sources of zinc include wheat germ, collard greens, cocoa, and oysters.

Did you know? Don't be fooled by labels that state "Natural Flavors." This is a vague term that can even mean a synthetic additive. Here's another great reason to eat whole foods: They are what they are.

Soaking and Sprouting

Legumes, nuts, seeds, and whole grains are awesome sources of nutrition. Think of them as little factories just waiting to have the lights turned on so they can begin manufacturing life energy. However, the same natural elements that protect them from early germination can make them difficult to digest and can impede our ability to absorb their nutrients.

Soaking and sprouting replicates germination, which activates multiple nutrients, neutralizes enzyme inhibitors, and promotes the activity of digestive enzymes. Sounds tricky, but it's so easy to do! To soak, dump the nuts/seeds/legumes into a glass container, cover with warm filtered water in a 2:1 water-to-seed ratio, and leave them alone overnight. Let them dry—they will crisp back up nicely.

Sprouting takes a couple days, but requires little effort for an enormous nutritional payoff. Check out sproutpeople.org to learn more about sprouting and how to get started.

DAILY
Building Blocks

The table below contains a summary of the Institute of Medicine's most current Dietary Reference Intake (DRI) in Pregnancy and Lactation of major nutrients for an average-weight adult female. Some experts and organizations may recommend more or less of a given nutrient. You may have slightly different needs. If your dietary intake comes from whole foods and is pretty consistent with the requirements listed in this table, you're on the right track.

KEY NUTRIENT	DAILY REQUIREMENT IN PREGNANCY/ LACTATION	WHAT IT DOES	WHERE TO GET IT	
Water	About 12 eight-ounce glasses	Assists in nearly every physiologic function	Fresh fruits and veggies, filtered water stored in glass	
Carbohydrates	175g/210g	Gives you usable energy for life	Fruits, vegetables, whole grains	
Protein	71g/71g	Needed for growth, cell division, immune function	Nuts, seeds, legumes, whole grains, organic dairy products, eggs, meats, wild fish	
Fats	500mg omega-3 fatty acids EPA and DHA (at least 300mg of this from DHA)	Makes up the cell membrane, important in all growth and development, hormone synthesis	Nuts, seeds, avocado, coconut, wild fatty fish, organic eggs	

KEY NUTRIENT	DAILY REQUIREMENT IN PREGNANCY/ LACTATION	WHAT IT DOES	WHERE TO GET IT	
Fiber	28g/29g	Feeds the good gut bacteria, keeps stool soft and bulky, prevents constipation	A variety of fruits, vegetables, whole grains	
Probiotics*	Minimum 10 billion live organisms	Maintains healthy gut microflora, prevents yeast infections and bacterial vaginosis, improves digestion and immune system function	Cultured and fermented foods, high-quality probiotic supplements	
Vitamin A	770mcg/1300mcg	Assists in organ development, fat metabolism, healing and tissue repair, vision	Carrots, iceberg lettuce, sweet potatoes, mangos, kale, cantaloupe	
Vitamin B$_6$	1.6mg/1.7mg	Involved in brain development and immune system function	Sunflower seeds, pistachio nuts, prunes, wild salmon, bananas, avocados, chickpeas	
Vitamin B$_7$ (Biotin)	30mcg/35mcg	Assists in metabolizing carbs, fats, and proteins, normal immune function, healthy hair and skin	Mushrooms, avocados, Swiss chard, berries, raw shelled sunflower seeds, eggs	
Vitamin B$_9$ (Folate)	600mcg/500mcg	Prevents birth defects (especially related to the nervous system), needed for cell division	Dark leafy greens (kale, collards, spinach), whole grains, legumes	
Vitamin B$_{12}$	2.6mcg/2.8mcg	Helps with brain and nervous system development, needed to absorb folate and choline	Tempeh, nutritional yeast, spirulina, organic eggs, wild fish	

*Probiotics are not included in the Institute of Medicine's Dietary Reference Intake tables but many studies show that they are highly beneficial (see References).

CONTINUED >>

DAILY BUILDING BLOCKS, CONTINUED

KEY NUTRIENT	DAILY REQUIREMENT IN PREGNANCY/ LACTATION	WHAT IT DOES	WHERE TO GET IT	
Vitamin C	85mg/120mg	Maintains healthy skin and connective tissues, collagen synthesis, immune function	Strawberries, papaya, broccoli, Brussels sprouts, bell peppers, guavas	
Vitamin D	600 IU/600 IU	Helps with bone and teeth development, immune function	Sunlight, organic egg yolks, fatty fish, sardines	
Vitamin K	90mcg/90mcg	Important for blood clotting, synthesis of protein in bones, plasma, and kidneys	Avocado, kale, collards, mustard greens, Brussels sprouts	
Zinc	11mg/12mg	Needed for protein and DNA synthesis, optimal immune function	Raw pepitas (shelled raw pumpkin seeds), wheat germ, almonds, collard greens, cocoa, oysters	
Choline	450mg/550mg	Assists in brain development, neurotransmitter synthesis, prevents neural tube defects	Soymilk, tofu, quinoa, broccoli, eggs, scallops	
Iron	27mg/9mg	Needed for hemoglobin to transport oxygen	Lentils, dark chocolate, dried peaches and prunes, cooked spinach, blackstrap molasses	
Copper	1000mcg/1300mcg	Needed for collagen synthesis, cofactor needed to incorporate iron into hemoglobin	Sesame seeds, cashews, soybeans, shiitake and crimini mushrooms, turnip greens	

KEY NUTRIENT	DAILY REQUIREMENT IN PREGNANCY/ LACTATION	WHAT IT DOES	WHERE TO GET IT	
Selenium	60mcg/70mcg	Provides antioxidant protection, normal thyroid function	Shiitake and crimini mushrooms, asparagus, sardines	
Magnesium	360mg/320mg	Important for healthy bowel function, muscle relaxation, bone health	Raw spinach, squash and pumpkin seeds, soybeans and lentils, dark chocolate, avocados	
Calcium	1000mg/1000mg	Ensures healthy bones and teeth, cardiovascular function	Fortified almond or soy milk, broccoli, tofu, bok choy, Chinese cabbage, organic dairy products	
Phosphorus	700mg/700mg	Needed for musculoskeletal system formation and function, heart rhythm	Soybeans, raw pepitas (shelled pumpkin seeds), scallops, sardines	
Iodine	220mcg/290mcg	Vital to thyroid hormone production	Sea vegetables (kelp, arame, hiziki, kombu), scallops, cod	
Potassium	4.7g/5.1g	Helps maintain normal blood pressure, kidney health, electrolyte and fluid balance	Beet greens, lima beans, Swiss chard, sweet potatoes, bok choy, spinach	

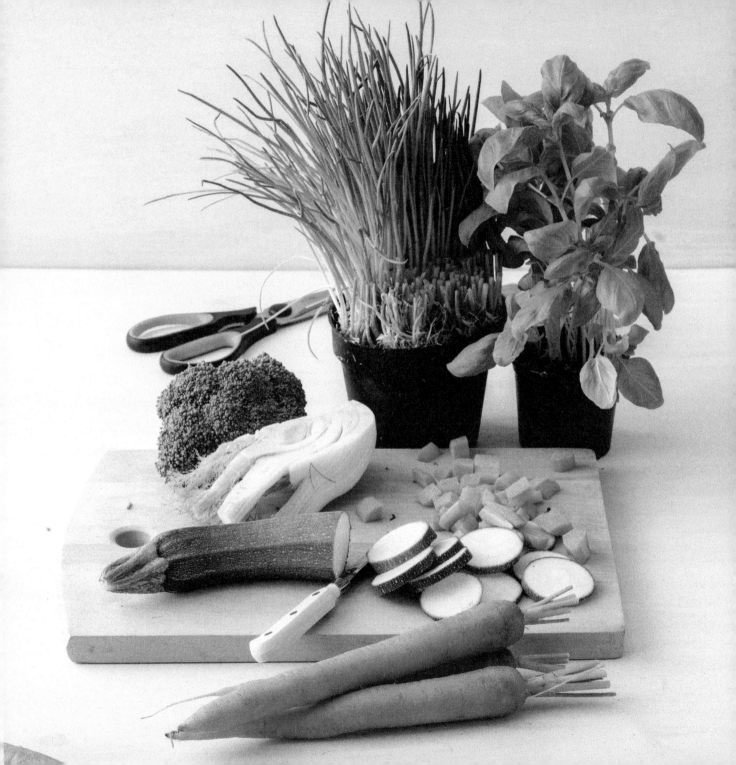

Part Two

PREGNANCY, WEEK BY WEEK

The information presented in part 1 of this book is a great blueprint for a healthy diet in pregnancy and beyond. We examined key nutrients needed for the healthy growth and development of your baby, reviewed basic guidelines for weight gain in each trimester, and addressed some common symptoms and side effects of pregnancy and dietary means for treating them. Now let's focus on the miracles happening in your baby's developing body from week to week during your entire pregnancy, and explore specific foods that will target, support, and nourish these changes.

three

FIRST TRIMESTER

· ·

The way a pregnancy is dated can be a little confusing. Unless you've undergone in vitro fertilization and the exact date of the embryo transfer is known, most pregnancies are dated from the LMP (last menstrual period). This date is the calendar date of the first day you started bleeding in your last period before getting pregnant. The due date is actually 40 weeks from the LMP. The trimesters are based on this date range. Because most women ovulate at about the middle of their four-week cycle, this means that the baby doesn't actually exist during the first two weeks of the first trimester. Strange, I know. Welcome to the fascinating world of pregnancy!

MONTH 1
WEEKS 1 TO 4

Many women are in a state of surprise or even shock during month 1. These emotions are normal—this is a life-changing event!

In month 1 you may not even know if you are pregnant. In this case, one of two basic scenarios will likely be taking place.

Scenario A: You have been trying to optimize your body for pregnancy, perhaps by eliminating big toxin exposures such as high blood sugar levels, alcohol, cigarettes, and prescription or nonprescription drugs. You might be taking supplemental folate or folic acid or you are working to get this from your diet.

Scenario B: You've been engaging in some nonoptimal but normal behaviors—and perhaps pregnancy is a surprise. While Scenario A is preferable, Scenario B happens often and generally is not consequential if mom gets on board with healthy habits.

Pregnant or not, treat your body like the gorgeous, sacred temple it is, and only put good things into it. While our modern world isn't always conducive to that approach, the best defense is a good offense. So use this month to begin arming yourself with information, and plan ahead for the foods you want in your home and in your body.

Week by Week

WEEK 1   You have your period. If you are trying to get pregnant, think positively: This may be your last week of tampons for a very long time!

WEEK 2   Enjoy a sensual week. The primary follicle developing and preparing to release the egg that meets the sperm and becomes your little beloved is working its pregestational magic right now. This is your week to have lots of amazing sex, and focus on feeling happy and relaxed so your body knows it's a good time to procreate. Toward the end of this week, most women are ovulating.

WEEK 3   Sperm has met egg, magic has happened, and we have a zygote. This zygote then divides into a blastocyst, which continues to divide as it makes its way down the fallopian tube. Toward the end of this week, the embryo picks a yummy, cushy spot on the wall of your uterus, where it will set up house for the next nine months.

How Big Is Baby?

WEEK 4. . . . . ⅛ INCH

WEEK 4 The embryo has implanted into the uterus, and the placenta is beginning to form, which is the incredibly important structure that will supply the baby with oxygen and nutrients for the remainder of its stay. Think of the placenta as a giant whole-house filtration system. The cells of the embryo, which is only the size of a poppy seed, are beginning to become specialized in their ultimate jobs of being a brain cell or heart cell or kidney cell. Most over-the-counter pregnancy tests will not be positive until the end of this week, so it is likely you don't even know you are pregnant.

FAQ

What if I'm overweight right now? Can I start a diet in pregnancy?
Don't think of it as a diet. Think of it as a change in lifestyle. If you are starting off in pregnancy with a body mass index that is obese (greater than 30; visit heart.org for their BMI calculator), you actually do not need to gain any weight during pregnancy as long as your fetus is growing appropriately. If you provide the right healthy foods, your fat stores will make up for the rest. No calorie counting, denial, or starvation is necessary. If you choose good foods, you can eat as much as you want, and you will be healthy.

What's on Your Plate?

Important nutrients at this point in your brand-new pregnancy include choline, vitamin B_{12}, folate/folic acid, and zinc. See pages 44–47 for foods containing these key nutrients. The following recipes were designed with your current needs in mind.

- EGGS AND GREENS (PAGE 96)
- POMEGRANATE GUACAMOLE (PAGE 122)
- PARSLEY PESTO PASTA (PAGE 176)
- TWO-BEAN SALAD (PAGE 142)
- QUICK AND EASY MINESTRONE (PAGE 132)

Every woman in my family gained at least 50 pounds in pregnancy, and their bodies were never the same again. Can I do it differently?
Yes, you can! Begin today, educate yourself through resources like this book, and follow through with mindful food decisions, and you can be in better shape post-pregnancy than you've ever been before.

WHAT'S IN A
Prenatal Vitamin?

A good prenatal vitamin is an excellent insurance policy against deficiency in any essential nutrient. Prenatal vitamins should not replace healthy eating, but just complement it. If you are planning to become pregnant, you may want to begin taking a prenatal vitamin prior to conception. This will give your body the best chance of having everything it needs for those earliest developmental processes. Recommended formulas should contain:

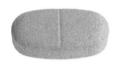

Calcium
Essential for building bones as well as teeth, heart, muscles, and nerves.

Choline
Protects newborns against neural tube defects.

Copper
In pregnancy, your blood supply increases and copper is essential for forming red blood cells.

Folate
For a healthy nervous system, heart, mouth, and brain.

Iodine
Helps in the development of your baby's brain and nervous system.

Magnesium
Assists in building and repairing your body's tissues as well as forming your baby's bones and teeth.

Phosphorus
Helps build strong bones in you and your baby.

Selenium
With antioxidant properties, it's crucial for thyroid health.

The B vitamins
Including B_5 (pantothenic acid), B_6 (pyridoxine), B_{12} (cobalamin), riboflavin, niacin, thiamine, biotin, important for a healthy nervous system.

Vitamins C, D, E
For healthy muscles and immune system, especially in helping the body absorb iron and calcium.

Zinc
Assists in supporting the immune system and healing wounds.

NOTES: Vitamins from whole-food sources are recommended. Also, some prenatal vitamins contain omega-3 fatty acids (EPA and DHA); if yours doesn't contain these, an additional supplement is recommended.

Vitamin brands can submit their products for testing to ensure that they meet the highest standards of quality and reliably contain what they say. Look for the seal of one of these trusted organizations: United States Pharmacopia (USP), Consumer Lab, or NSF International.

MONTH 2
WEEKS 5 TO 8

Month 2 is pretty much the beginning of pregnancy from your perspective. If you were one of the moms in month 1's scenario B, you may find yourself worried because you ingested some toxins. I hope that some kind soul gave you this book to read so you can take a breath and let it go. What is past, is past. Now that you know you are pregnant, you can stop ingesting the very bad things, cut down substantially on the "kind-of" bad things, and significantly increase your intake of the great things.

Months 2 and 3 can be some of the most mind-boggling of pregnancy. You may still be wrapping your head around the idea of becoming a mother, and that head is probably already spinning with a million abstract thoughts about the future. But these months are also an incredible opportunity to plan, dream, and, of course, make shifts in your entire system of self-care that will have a tremendous positive impact on your life and your family's generations to come.

Week by Week

WEEK 5 This week you may have noticed your period has not arrived. Maybe you ran to the pharmacy and grabbed a two-pack of pee sticks. Seeing a positive pregnancy test can be a very emotional moment. It is normal to have conflicting feelings, especially if you haven't been especially pristine with your self-care over the past few weeks. Don't worry. Just get yourself a prenatal vitamin containing folate, vitamin B_{12}, and choline, and start taking it so your baby, who's currently the size of a peppercorn, can start reaping the rewards.

If you smoke cigarettes or marijuana, please stop, and stop drinking alcohol. If you find this is hard for you, or you feel like you can't, please seek treatment with an addiction specialist immediately. (A listing of specialists in your area can be found on the American Society of Addiction Medicine's website, or asam.org.) A specialist will not judge you, but rather commend and support you for this incredibly courageous decision. The benefit of getting clean and sober for both you and your baby is immeasurable.

This week is a great opportunity to focus on foods rich in the essential nutrients folate, vitamin B_{12}, and choline, which help in organ system development (see pages 44–47).

How Big Is Baby?

WEEK 5 . . . . ⅙ INCH

WEEK 6 . . . . ¼ INCH

WEEK 7 . . . . ½ INCH

WEEK 8 . . . . ⅝ INCH

WEEK 6   Your baby looks like a tiny fish, complete with embryonic tail! An immature but basic heart is now beating, pumping blood throughout your baby's body and supplying all the key ingredients her newly developing organ systems need to grow. The neural tube (from which the brain and spinal column form) fully closes by the end of this week, so do your best to get those important key nutrients in by diet or supplement, or both.

Your breasts may feel fuller than normal, and slightly sore. You may have occasional nausea or notice that you have become sensitive to certain smells. You may feel more tired than usual. Tapering down or eliminating caffeine intake will help with breast tenderness and sleep quality. If you've tried tapering down on the wine and you can't, and find yourself justifying it by saying things like, "But in Europe they drink wine," please call that addiction specialist you didn't call last week. *Alcohol is the greatest cause of preventable birth defects in the United States.* (For more information or to find a specialist in your area, visit the American Society of Addiction Medicine's website, or asam.org.)

Regular exercise is also important and can help significantly with nausea. Just don't go above an 8 on the "perceived exertion scale" (see chart on page 25) and stay well hydrated with water and electrolytes if needed.

WEEK 7   Little limb buds are beginning to sprout from the sides of baby's body, which will grow into his arms and legs. At this stage of development, we really do look like the primordial creatures you might imagine crawling out of the oceans to colonize the earth. The magical sound of baby's heartbeat is usually detectable on ultrasound beginning at some point this week.

Even though your baby is only the size of a blueberry, the basic framework for almost all major organs and body parts has been set by this week. Now it's just a matter of nourishing them to grow into their optimal potential. Do your best with nutrient-rich whole foods, but if you are battling nausea and can't stomach much besides crackers (whole grain of course, preferably with some seeds), remember the message in part 1 of this book: *It is more important in the first trimester for you to avoid ingesting toxins than it is to take in nutrients for your baby's development.* Just stay well hydrated with sips of nonsugary liquids, and try to keep down your prenatal vitamin to cover your nutritional bases.

WEEK 8   Your baby's embryonic tail is starting to disappear, and her limbs look less like knobs on a tree and more like arms and legs. The heart is now beating strongly and blood is circulating throughout the body, even filtering through developing kidneys. Coincidentally, baby is now the size of a kidney bean.

Nausea and vomiting may take on more of a prominent role in your life, but some cardiovascular exercise will help alleviate that issue. This is about the week in my first pregnancy when I perfected the art of mouth-breathing to avoid smells in the operating room, and prepared for each surgery by packing my waistline with ice to fend off nausea. We adapt. It's what we were made to do!

Also, try bland whole foods containing electrolytes and some extra vitamin B6. Bananas, potatoes, and raw shelled sunflower seeds are good options.

FAQ

I feel so sick! Should I take antinausea drugs?
There are lists of prescription drugs commonly prescribed during pregnancy in the past that we now know are associated with harmful effects in the developing baby. When it comes to drugs, I'm a minimalist. Ginger in any form or peppermint tea can help greatly with nausea. If you cannot keep down sips of liquids, have tried and exhausted all the tips and tricks to help with nausea, have tried and failed acupuncture and/or acupressure, and have documented electrolyte imbalances from dehydration, only then would I consider using the lowest dose of a drug recommended by your obstetrician for the shortest duration necessary.

What's on Your Plate?

This month, you and baby rely on organ development foods: folate, choline, vitamin B12, potassium, magnesium, phosphorus, and vitamin B6. See pages 44–47 for foods that provide these elements. The following recipes also pay special attention to these key nutrients.

- BANANA-WALNUT SMOOTHIE BOWL (PAGE 103)
- TROPICAL FRUIT SALAD (PAGE 118)
- CURRIED SQUASH (PAGE 153)
- WILD RICE SALAD (PAGE 143)
- GINGER-LEMONGRASS BROTH (PAGE 129)

I'm sick every day. The only things I can eat right now are saltine crackers and ginger ale. Is my baby going to be okay?
Think of your baby as a beautiful little sponge that lives in your womb. It will pretty much take what it needs from you. If you are not taking in enough good nutrition in the first trimester, it's likely to be you who suffers more, with your body's stores depleted. Check in with your obstetrician regularly, and try to get your prenatal vitamins in; taking them at bedtime can alleviate the nausea that sometimes follows. (For antinausea remedies, see the list on page 57).

When You Don't Want to Eat

Some women find that having a little something in their stomach early in the day has a settling effect. Some women don't, and that's fine too. We figure out what works best for us, and when it doesn't work anymore, we adapt. Sometimes it's not a food that provides the fix—applying ice to the mouth, face, or neck can also bring quick relief. Find your solution and exploit it in every way.

Combine some of the suggestions below. Try making banana-ginger "ice cream" by mixing these two ingredients in a blender, then freezing the mixture immediately.

Citrus

The smell of citrus is reported by many women to help with nausea. Dab a tiny drop of orange essential oil above your upper lip. Squeeze a lemon into a tall glass of ice water and sip throughout the day. Instead of beginning each day with coffee or tea, try hot water and lemon for its myriad benefits (including antinausea).

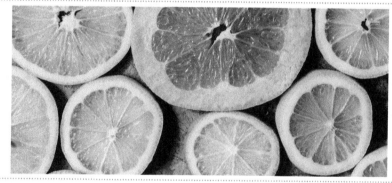

Ginger

Ginger is the number-one food for battling nausea. Boil fresh whole or sliced peeled ginger root in hot water and sip the tea—it's a powerful treatment for morning sickness. Some women like the crunch of pickled ginger, others like the sweet of a candied ginger chew (just go light on these if they contain sugar or other sweeteners).

Foods with B_6

Bananas, carrots, spinach, sunflower seeds, pineapple, and avocados are all healthy sources of vitamin B_6, a nutrient shown to be helpful in preventing nausea during pregnancy.

Bland foods

Try simple whole foods that include fiber to clear chemicals from your system, like brown rice, baked potatoes, broth, brown rice crackers, and plain whole grain pasta.

MONTH 3
WEEKS 9 TO 13

Most women know whether they are pregnant by month 3. If you suddenly realize you have now missed not one, but two periods, now is a great time to do a pregnancy test.

Reflect on your body, the sacred temple housing mom and her growing baby. Taking care of yourself has never resulted in greater rewards. Bring good things into your life and let go of what you don't need. This may mean taking a nap in the middle of the day. This may mean ending your love affair with Diet Coke. Perhaps treat yourself to your first prenatal massage.

Your emotions can affect how your body is feeling. Anxiety, for one, worsens nausea. You may take medication for anxiety, but since you are pregnant, substitutions are sometimes required. During this time of new discoveries, consider the myriad benefits of a mindfulness-based meditation practice. Do a web search on the subject, read up on the basics, and start with just five minutes a day. Meditation involves simple things, like focus, conscious breathing, and gentle movements, and it can really help your clarity of thinking and perspective (among other benefits). In fact, it can alleviate many pregnancy-related symptoms and help you maintain a healthier diet and general outlook.

Week by Week

WEEK 9 The embryonic tail has disappeared completely by the end of this week, and baby is definitely more human looking, although only the size of a grape. Organs continue to grow and develop, becoming increasingly functional and specialized in their activities.

This is peak nausea time for most women who experience this malady in pregnancy. Go heavy on the fluids and electrolytes, and take frequent small bites of bland foods. Getting sufficient exercise and high-quality sleep can make a huge difference in the way you feel. You will get through this. You're a mother now—you can do anything.

WEEK 10 The baby's neck begins to develop this week, taste buds are forming on her little tongue, and eyelids are growing to cover and protect the developing eyes. The embryonic phase of development ends at the completion of this week,

How Big Is Baby?

WEEK 9	¾ INCH
WEEK 10	1 INCH*
WEEK 11	1½ INCHES
WEEK 12	2 INCHES
WEEK 13	3 INCHES
WEEK 13 WEIGHT	1 OUNCE

*Crown-to-rump length from Week 10 to Week 20

which means your baby will officially be considered a fetus. I hope your meditation practice is in full swing, because you are now one developmental step closer to having a toddler.

Your baby is about the size of a prune, a good fruit to think about at this point if you are suffering from constipation. Lots of warm liquids and some dried fruit can really help here. You might also consider avoiding a meat-heavy diet, which is highly constipating.

WEEK 11 Your baby now has genitals and has started to pee. Isn't that cute? I'm trying to give you something fun to hold onto, because pregnancy right around now may not feel so fun. If you have experienced morning sickness, it's likely been going on for a few weeks in a row, and you might be wondering if you will ever feel like yourself again (you will).

Developmentally, your baby's ears have also appeared, set low on the baby's head, and muscle tissue is beginning to form throughout the body.

WEEK 12 Your baby is now producing and swallowing little sips of amniotic fluid. A four-chambered heart is efficiently pumping oxygen and nutrient-rich blood around the body to feed the developing parts. Bones and cartilage are being built, and increased muscle mass means your baby is now going to start moving a little more vigorously (though you won't quite feel it yet), stretching her little limbs and kicking her little future soccer-playing feet. Baby fingernails also make their debut this week.

What's on Your Plate?

At this stage of development, try to get plenty of fiber, magnesium, potassium, and zinc to counter some of the side effects you may be experiencing. See the table on pages 44–47 for foods to include, and try out the following nutritionally rich recipes.

- AVOCADO TOAST (PAGE 96)
- WILD WATERMELON COOLER (PAGE 121)
- BANANA-COCONUT BITES (PAGE 124)
- COBB PASTA SALAD (PAGE 147)
- TOFU STIR-FRY (PAGE 162)

WEEK 13 Unique little fingerprints have developed on the tips of your baby's fingers. Arms and legs are moving about, and sometimes an ultrasound will show the beginning of thumb-sucking. The intestines, which up to this point have been located inside the umbilical cord, begin to move inside the abdomen. The baby's vocal chords are beginning to develop (you will one day come to intimately recognize the sound emitted from these structures). Testes are producing testosterone in males, and ovaries are rapidly producing eggs in females (yes, already!). Essentially your baby is on a total roll and you, Mama, are making it all possible.

Congratulations—you just conquered your first trimester!

FAQ

I haven't been eating well or taking care of myself. Have I done permanent damage to my baby?

Babies are remarkably tenacious and incredibly resilient. They compensate very well for sub-optimal conditions during a limited portion of their growth and development. They are also greedy and take what they need out of you, even if it means depleting your health. Look to the future and begin caring for yourself today. Every day that you eat well and engage in nurturing behaviors will benefit both you and your baby.

I've read about gluten being detrimental during pregnancy. Should I follow a gluten-free diet?

"Gluten" is a name given to the protein in wheat, rye, barley, and oats that people with celiac disease react to. Peer-reviewed research shows that gluten causes a weakening in the tight-junctions of the gut mucosa in everyone (not just people with celiac disease or gluten sensitivity). Since this "leakiness" of the gut mucosa permits incompletely digested molecules' entry into circulation, where there is increased potential for an immune reaction and inflammation, it may be reasonable to attempt to reduce or eliminate gluten from our diets.

If you are following a whole-foods diet, you are well on your way to being gluten-free without even trying. Whole fruits and vegetables, nuts, seeds, and legumes do not contain gluten. Neither do the grains or "pseudo-grains" (which are seeds, not grains) in the following list. Soaking or sprouting (see page 43) or even fermenting (see Resources) pseudo-grains ramps up their nutritional value.

- **GLUTEN-CONTAINING:** barley, bulgur, couscous, durum, farro, kamut, oats, rye, semolina, spelt, wheat

- **GLUTEN-FREE:** acacia (wattle seed), amaranth, buckwheat, chia, corn, millet, rice, quinoa, sorghum, wild rice

Folate-Rich
FOODS

Folate, also called vitamin B9, is found in nature and is protective against neural tube defects during early fetal development. Folic acid is a synthetic equivalent used to supplement the diet in vitamins and fortified foods. Most of this vitamin should come from whole foods. Twelve foods high in folate include:

Asparagus		Lentils
Black beans		Mustard greens
Broccoli		Pinto beans
Collard greens		Romaine lettuce
Edamame		Spinach
Garbanzo beans		Turnip greens

four

SECOND TRIMESTER

Many women love their second trimester of pregnancy. You've had a little time to adjust to the idea of being pregnant. You've hopefully made an honest start at eliminating some avoidable toxins from your lifestyle. You've used some pregnancy tips that have helped with classic first-trimester symptoms, and now your body seems to be starting to cooperate (and maybe also to grow). That classic "pregnancy glow" may be emerging, fatigue and nausea abating, and for a good part of the second trimester, you can probably still wear your regular jeans. What's not to love? Read on and love it more by learning what extraordinary transformations are going on inside you.

MONTH 4
WEEKS 14 TO 17

By month 4, you have likely established regular prenatal care with an OB/GYN or midwife. They are hopefully giving you information and guidance on nutrition and self-care in pregnancy, as well as general weight gain recommendations.

If you began your pregnancy at a normal weight (based on BMI; see table on page 35), from this point on in the pregnancy, you can expect to gain about 1 pound a week. If your pre-pregnancy weight fell into the overweight BMI category, you need to gain less, and if it was in the obese category, you do not need to gain any weight at all. Stepping on the scale naked on Monday mornings after you have peed and writing down the number is not being crazy or obsessive. Doing it daily is not the best idea, though. Your body fluctuates from day to day, and can vary by up to five pounds just from water retention. A weekly weigh-in is a healthy and natural way of keeping track and not veering far from your goal. If watching the numbers on the scale slowly increase is particularly distressing for you, consider a consultation with a whole-foods nutritionist who specializes in eating disorders who can help you decide if you might benefit from additional support.

Most of the information in this book is written assuming a singleton pregnancy. If you are going to have twins, triplets, or more, you will need to gain more weight and have special nutrient needs (see page 39).

Week by Week

WEEK 14 Your baby's body is now starting to catch up with the size of his head, and the result is a more proportionate-looking fetus. His arms and legs are growing longer and more proportionate to the body as well. The brain has divided into two hemispheres, and the baby can begin to react to external stimuli. Even rudimentary facial expressions can be detected starting this week.

You may be noticing changes in your own body, such as a deepening in the color of your nipples or even your labia. Some women need to up-size their bra around this point in pregnancy. Your hair and nails may appear thicker and healthier—thanks, prenatal vitamins!

How Big Is Baby?

WEEK 14	3½ INCHES
WEEK 15	4 INCHES
WEEK 16	4½ INCHES
WEEK 17	5 INCHES
WEEK 17 WEIGHT	5 OUNCES

The second trimester is when you may need to begin to consume a few extra calories each day to keep up with your baby's growth. This will usually happen naturally, as you start to move away from the nausea of early pregnancy and your appetite tends to improve. Apply these extra calories wisely. Your baby relies on you to provide the good stuff it can build with. Remember to eat the rainbow! If you fill up on colorful and fiber-filled whole foods with lots of phytonutrients, you will find it's actually challenging to gain fat.

WEEK 15 What? Yes, your baby's ears have now begun to transmit sounds to the brain, so if you're not already, go ahead and start talking and singing softly to your baby—she can hear you! Bones all over her body are going through a process of ossification, or hardening. The spinal cord is fully formed by the end of this week. Your baby has also started manufacturing her own fat cells, which she can harness to create her own energy, although she continues to obtain all the glucose and fatty acids she needs through the placenta. Stores of a kind of fat called brown fat have begun to accumulate, which, along with lanugo (a fine coat of hair), blanket your little treasure to provide insulation and warmth.

What's on Your Plate?

This month, you and your baby can benefit from a boost in calcium, vitamin D, and magnesium. Foods with these nutrients are listed on pages 44–47, and are also present in abundance in the following recipes.

- TOFU SCRAMBLE (PAGE 102)
- AVOCADO-HEMP SPREAD (PAGE 125)
- ROASTED TOFU RICE BOWLS (PAGE 179)
- ARUGULA SALAD (PAGE 144)
- VEGGIE KEBAB (PAGE 185)

WEEK 16 Your baby is continuing his phenomenal growth spurt. In the next few weeks he will double in size. Toenails develop now, and those little legs are stretching and kicking up a storm (though you probably can't feel it yet). The eyes have moved even closer together toward the front of the face, and the ears have almost arrived at their permanent position on the head.

WEEK 17 The umbilical cord is thickening and strengthening, becoming a freeway populated by virtual Mack trucks of nutrients supplying oxygen and developmental building blocks and removing carbon dioxide and waste materials for mama to excrete. Yes, you've already started cleaning up after your baby.

When I think about how all of this happens so naturally and continuously without us even needing to think about it, it really is remarkably convenient. This won't last forever—before you know it, you'll be manually changing her diapers, cooking and clearing her dishes, and picking up her toys off the playroom floor—but that's special in its own way, too.

FAQ

What kinds of sushi and sashimi can I eat?
Avoid sushi for two reasons. (1) Consuming uncooked fish increases risk for a food-borne bacterial or parasitic infection. Just a few offenders are salmon, trout, pike, seabass, cod, herring mackerel, squid, crab, yellowfin tuna, oysters, and clams. Cooking these fish decreases the risk of ingesting live parasites or larvae. (2) Certain fish higher up the food chain can bioaccumulate toxins to which fetuses, infants, and young children are particularly sensitive. In particular, avoid farmed salmon and bluefin tuna.

My heartburn is really annoying and uncomfortable. I feel like TUMS is making up most of my diet these days. What else can I take?
The elevated progesterone from your pregnancy relaxes the sphincters that keep parts of the digestive tract where they are supposed to be. Gastric emptying time is also delayed, keeping food in the stomach longer than usual. Additionally, your growing uterus is starting to press upward on the stomach, decreasing the amount of physical space in there. These factors allow for a lot more reflux to come up into the esophagus, causing heartburn. TUMS and similar antacids are basically candied chalk that absorb and neutralize stomach acid. You need stomach acid in order to digest your food, properly absorb nutrients, and move food through your system. Antacids do nothing to address the underlying issue. Instead, refer to the section on managing heartburn (see page 22) for healthy tips that get to the root cause.

Substitutes

Pregnancy is famous for causing women to experience cravings. When a craving strikes, think about it. Are you craving something because you forgot to eat and your blood sugar is plummeting? Are you really hungry, or is this hunger more emotional, and you just need some noncaloric TLC? Perhaps you are not hungry but thirsty; have a glass of water. Are you in fact tired, and the cortisol spike is triggering a sugar craving? Sometimes we just need to shut the refrigerator door and our mind, and lie down.

Occasionally we really do want some sugar, fat, or salt. The trick is to find these things in natural, whole-food sources, and combine them with some fiber and protein to make them satisfying and keep you satiated longer. If you have a real craving, try substituting these delicious and nourishing choices for the empty-calorie antinutrient alternatives.

WANT THIS	TRY THIS
Chocolate	Good-quality dark chocolate or organic chocolate milk
Diet Coke	Filtered water with sliced fruit or sugar-free seltzer water, if desired
French fries	Hand-cut baked sweet potato fries
Pizza	Homemade pizza with sautéed veggies and sauce on a whole wheat crust sprinkled with Parmesan cheese
Cookies	Homemade cookies with nuts and/or seeds
Ice cream	Scoop of organic ice cream with lots of nuts and berries on top
Pickles	Kimchi, sauerkraut, or miso
Fruit juice	Fresh fruit or raw veggie juice sweetened with carrot or apple juice
Potato chips and onion dip	Carrot sticks and hummus

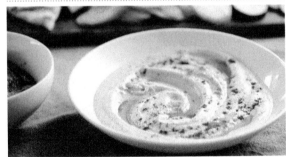

MONTH 5
WEEKS 18 TO 22

Month 5 is a busy one; a lot is happening to you and within you. Most women will have a little bump now, and many of you will make the shift to maternity clothes. Thankfully, those clothes have gotten so much cuter than they were years ago. So love your bump! Show off your bump! You are glowing and active and healthy, and the epitome of gestating gorgeousness.

A fascinating thing that happens to most women in month 5 is the distinct sensation of another being moving inside, independent of your body. Week 18 is usually the earliest that women will feel this sensation, called quickening. When you feel it for the first time, you may gasp—it is such an utterly foreign sensation. You may have been singing or talking to your baby for a while now, but this is your baby's first real communication with *you*. There's no denying it

now: baby's here and very real. Yep, if you need a concrete sensation to remind you to make healthy food choices, month 5 will give it to you.

Week by Week

WEEK 18 All five of baby's senses are now developed, so continue to talk and sing to her. This was the week when (as an exuberant pregnant obstetrician) I started religiously wearing a band around my abdomen that played progressively more complex percussive sounds, purportedly designed to stimulate the baby's brain development.

At this time in development, your baby's nerves are being optimized for effective transmission—this process benefits from lots of healthy plant fats and proteins. Respond to this need by taking in some nice fresh avocado and some seeds and nuts.

WEEK 19 The kidneys continue to make baby urine, which forms the amniotic fluid that fills the amniotic sac to make the little swimming pool your baby enjoys throughout pregnancy (don't be put off by this image—the body is a miracle filter, and your baby is quite safe and content). The flavors of what you eat make their way into this pool, and your baby now has both the taste buds and the neurological bandwidth to experience them.

As the nausea of the first trimester is generally resolved by this point, now is a great time to branch out in your dietary flavor repertoire. Not

---

How Big Is Baby?

WEEK 18	5½ INCHES
WEEK 19	6 INCHES
WEEK 20	6½ INCHES
WEEK 21	10½ INCHES*
WEEK 21 WEIGHT	12 OUNCES

*Head-to-heel length from Week 21 to 41+

only will this help you diversify your diet, learn some new favorites, and maybe discover some different nutrients, but it's also a great way to introduce these new flavors to your baby.

Vernix, a waxy protective coating, is starting to be produced and cover the baby's skin. Normal human head-to-body-to-limb ratios are now apparent. Start paying attention when you first wake up in the morning, or when you lie down. You may feel the first fluttering of movement inside you.

WEEK 20 If pregnancy is like running a marathon, you have just reached the half-marathon mark. Woohoo!

Your baby is now only about a month away from being considered viable in the extreme case that he needs to exist outside your womb. The cells lining his intestines are now producing meconium, the black-colored gooey stuff that makes up your baby's first bowel movement. And more exciting, an ultrasound done this week can usually tell you the gender of your baby.

If you take the side of your thumb and press firmly inward a couple inches above your belly button, then stroke downward toward your pelvis, you will likely bump up against the top of your uterus, right about the level of your belly button, roughly 20 centimeters from your pubic bone. The distance between the top of your uterus and your pubic bone is the *fundal height* that your healthcare provider will start measuring to track fetal growth. If you can believe it,

it will increase by about 1 centimeter per week from this point onward (effectively dating your pregnancy).

With all this growth, keep up with your fluids, proteins, and iron-rich foods so you don't experience dizziness or anemia.

WEEK 21 Growth and development in every organ system marches onward as your baby's size and weight increase. She is now weighing in at about 12 ounces (or ¾ pound). As bone and teeth mineralization continues to occur (this week, your baby starts building her permanent chompers—the baby teeth already began development many weeks ago!), make sure your diet is filled with healthy sources of calcium, vitamin D, magnesium, and phosphorus.

On the subject of vitamin D, why not go sit in the sun for a little while? A recent study demonstrated that the children of women who sunbathed moderately during pregnancy had stronger bones. I am not convinced that vitamin D supplements are adequate to replace what I consider a chronic sunlight deficiency in modern society. Don't roast yourself red, but consider ten minutes of bare, unsunblocked skin exposure during peak UVB daylight hours.

Oh, and your baby's little eyebrows are starting to grow in. How sweet is that?

WEEK 22 The much-overlooked but incredibly essential organ we call the pancreas is going through a developmental surge. This organ is responsible for producing digestive enzymes that will help your baby break down and metabolize fats. It is also where insulin is produced to help your baby regulate and control his blood sugar levels.

So let's talk about *your* blood sugar levels. Your circulating maternal blood sugar level is setting up your baby in terms of what he expects to find in his environment once he is born, so the way you are eating will be modeled by your baby before you even realize you are being watched. Whole foods are not a culprit— eat all the apples, melons, and peaches you want to. It's the added sweeteners and processed foods you need to watch out for. If high blood sugar has been an issue for you before or during pregnancy, seek out some cherries and berries, which affect blood sugar less strongly than do other fruits.

Either way, get your natural sweet on with whole foods, and avoid adding sugar or sugar substitutes to your food. Aside from being better for your baby, maintaining good blood sugar levels reduces the likelihood that you will have to repeat those yucky glucose tolerance tests.

FAQ

What exactly are GMO foods? Are these foods okay to eat in pregnancy?

GMO, or "genetically modified organism," includes any organism whose DNA has been altered by genetic engineering. GMOs in our food supply generally refer to foods that have been altered to be resistant to pests directly, or resistant to the application of certain herbicides, which can then be sprayed liberally to kill the weeds without damaging the crop. Over 90 percent of the corn, soy, and sugar beets grown and sold in the United States come from GMO seed. Furthermore, dousing the earth with herbicides and pesticides destroys soil quality, and so the crops that grow out of depleted soil are depleted themselves.

I do not recommend GMO foods. I support GMO labeling laws so consumers can make their own decisions about whether they want to consume these foods. In the meantime, if you stick with foods labeled USDA organic, they will by definition be free of GMOs.

PREGNANCY
Superfoods

Superfoods is a term given to foods that pack an extraordinary nutritional punch and often contain health-supportive and preventive properties. Though not exhaustive, these are some foods that I consider worthy to wear a Superfood crown:

Avocados
Peel avocados carefully; much of the nutritients are concentrated close to the peel. Avocados are fatty, but it's a good fat, balanced by high levels of fiber, vitamin K, and more.

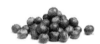

Bananas
Got a cramp? The potassium in bananas can help with those pesky leg cramps in pregnancy. Bananas also help with nausea and, over the long-term, with blood pressure and cholesterol.

Black beans
Toss these gems into your salad, meatloaf, or tacos for a varied vitamin boost and enhanced digestive health.

Blueberries
So much more than just a yummy treat, this antioxidant and anti-inflammatory power-house is loaded with nutrients.

Brussels sprouts
These nutrient-abundant little veggies are linked with cancer prevention. Three words for haters: Try them roasted (with lemon and sea salt).

Carrots
Good for the eyes, indeed (that's the vitamin A), and this readily available snack is associated with reduced risk for cardio-vascular disease.

Chia seeds
Sneak a spoonful of these into your oatmeal for a giant boost in fiber, omega-3s, and manganese.

Cucumbers
Anti-inflammatory, mild-tasting, and used tra-ditionally to help treat water retention and headaches. One of pregancy's perfect tools.

Garlic

Garlic is as good for you as it is delicious. Another healer, garlic fights heart disease and lowers cholesterol. Tip: Let it sit a bit after you chop it for maximum nutrition.

Green tea

Go green for its healing properties. Green tea is a powerful fighter of free radicals that try to hasten the aging process and alter DNA.

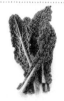

Leafy greens (mustard greens, spinach, kale, broccoli)

More decadent salad recipes are out there than ever before. Love your greens, and they will reward you with good health and disease prevention.

Pecans, walnuts, and/ or almonds

There may not be a better grab-and-go snack than nuts. Full of antioxidants and anti-inflammatory properties, they're a great source of sustained energy to boot.

Quinoa

If you haven't tried it yet, explore this anti-inflammatory, gluten-free food that will fill you up while providing loads of manganese, copper, and phosphorus.

Shiitake mushrooms

Pay a little extra for these special 'shrooms. In addition to their iron and protein, they fight viruses and infection and have anticancer properties.

For more information on these and other superfoods, visit whfoods.com.

MONTH 6
WEEKS 23 TO 27

Even beyond your pregnant glow, you likely look like an honest-to-goodness pregnant woman now. If you still can, this is probably the last month you will be able to get away with hiding your belly under a bulky sweater when you want to sneak onto an airplane without a note from your obstetrician.

This is also the month where you will cross the momentous and somewhat reassuring border of what the medical community refers to as "viability." At 23 weeks (when you enter your twenty-fourth week of gestation), the baby is considered able to survive outside of a mother's womb. But even though you've reached the viability marker, your baby's growth, and important developmental progressions will continue in the weeks to come.

How Big Is Baby?

WEEK 23	11 INCHES
WEEK 24	12 INCHES
WEEK 25	13½ INCHES
WEEK 26	14 INCHES
WEEK 27	14½ INCHES
WEEK 27 WEIGHT	2 POUNDS

You may have already found out whether it's a boy or a girl (if you wanted to know)—or perhaps both, if you're carrying multiples. Now the planning takes on a whole new meaning. Isn't it magical to dream about what's soon to come?

Week by Week

WEEK 23 Baby now probably weighs about a pound. This may seem small, but he is already as heavy as your one-pound bag of carrots—and he will double this weight over the next four weeks. The developing veins and arteries just beneath your baby's skin give him a reddish hue. You can still see the blood vessels, bones, and organs through his skin because the fatty layer that will ultimately surround the organs and plump up his skin hasn't caught up yet.

Stay active. Get outside and go for a vigorous hike in nature; just stay well hydrated when you do. Focus on walking, stretching, and getting good-quality sleep. Healthy plant fats and lots of vitamin C will help your skin stay healthy, supple, and radiant.

WEEK 24 This week is a key time for lung development in your baby. The cells in the lungs begin to manufacture surfactant (a slippery soap-like substance) this week, which is required to keep the little air sacs open and able to exchange oxygen for carbon dioxide. Maternal smoking or other nicotine use inhibits fetal lung development, and the effects persist into childhood. If you or your partner has not stopped smoking, please recruit whatever support you need and do so now. And keep your air intake fresh—keep a good distance from anyone who is smoking.

If you are carrying twins, it's time to think about the "24 pounds by 24 weeks" weight gain recommendation—you're here. How are you doing? If you are under this weight gain milestone, reach out for a consultation with a whole-foods nutritionist or your physician. If you're above, make sure your blood pressure is within normal range and that you don't have protein in your urine. Get that nutrition consult also, and dial down a bit on the calories. Explore and expand your culinary horizons. Look over the recipes in this book, wander your produce aisles, or visit your local local farmers' market.

At the end of this week, throw yourself a "viability party." Why not? I recommend getting in all the parties you can while you don't have to pay for a babysitter.

WEEK 25 A gymnast, already? Yes, your baby is developing a sense of balance and directional orientation, so lots of fun somersaults are happening in the play-pool of your amniotic sac. You will likely be feeling lots of movement, and may even be able to predict these movements as your baby acquires her own sleep-wake patterns.

What's on Your Plate?

Vitamin C, zinc, and vitamin A are your dietary buzzwords for this month. See pages 44–47 for whole-food ideas, and expand your culinary horizons with these tasty recipes that contain all the right nutritional elements.

- MANGO-BANANA SMOOTHIE (PAGE 105)
- REFRIGERATOR OATS (PAGE 106)
- AVOCADO AND BLACK BEAN SALAD (PAGE 148)
- KALE AND MANGO SALAD (PAGE 147)
- SIX-INGREDIENT CHILI (PAGE 139)

WEEK 26 Your voice and that of your partner are now clearly heard and recognized by your baby as nerves continue to grow in the ears and hearing centers of her brain. Practice saying kind and loving things—to yourself, to your partner, and to your baby. These messages get into your baby's brain, and they are transforming the hormonal atmosphere within your body to one that feels safe and happy for your baby.

A diet high in essential fatty acids and vitamin A is important for the neurocognitive development going on, including all this hearing.

WEEK 27 Your baby now sleeps and wakes, and can open and close his eyes when doing so. The irises are fully pigmented, though eye color can, and often does, continue to change even after birth. You may also become aware of your baby's hiccups, which are caused by involuntary contractions of the diaphragm as your baby practices taking little sips of amniotic fluid. Apparently, spicy foods can trigger fetal hiccups (expect about a two-hour delay from when you ate the food).

Continue to play with new flavors and spices. Many of these are filled with important nutrition. And remember, you are literally building the foundation for your baby's taste palate and preferences throughout his life.

Bravissima, mama! You've conquered the second trimester!

FAQ

Many of my relatives have Type 2 diabetes and I'm worried about developing gestational diabetes. Is there anything I can do to prevent this?

Yes! Foremost, do not gain more than the recommended amount of weight for your pre-pregnancy body mass index. If you were in the obese BMI category before pregnancy, you do not need to gain any weight at all. Also, eat a low-glycemic-index diet (foods that do not cause a rapid rise in blood sugar) and avoid processed grains and added sweeteners (even those zero-calorie non-nutritive options). A plant-based diet is considered the best choice for preventing diabetes. Fruits are fine, but always choose the whole fruit over the juice or dried fruit. Low-glycemic-index fruits like cherries and berries are best. You can add cinnamon to your meals to decrease their glycemic impact. Exercise daily with at least 20 to 30 minutes of an activity that elevates your heart rate. Just stay below a level 8 on the perceived exertion scale (see page 25).

GESTATIONAL DIABETES-FRIENDLY
Snacks

If you've been diagnosed with gestational diabetes, you may be wondering, What can I snack on and still be healthy? The answer is, so much! There are countless delicious foods out there waiting to be discovered and rediscovered. Try some of these great options that really satisfy you without tipping the sugar scales:

Almonds	**Cherries and berries** (some studies show that tart cherries aid in blood glucose control in diabetics)	
Apples	**Cinnamon** (when added to any food will decrease its glycemic impact)	
Bean or nut butter dips	Hard-boiled egg	
	Homemade guacamole	Raw carrot sticks
	Light popcorn	Raw sunflower and pumpkin seeds
	Raw, unsweetened almond, peanut, or cashew butters	Veggies and hummus

five

THIRD TRIMESTER

···························

Welcome to the home stretch! If you are in the position where maybe you have just gotten your hands on this book, and/or you may not have been eating the healthiest diet up to this point, don't despair! The third trimester clarifies again the importance of eating a whole-foods diet filled with lots of colorful plants. Baby is still developing and can benefit greatly from your good choices. As your belly grows and your weight begins to shift to the front of you, a healthy diet can also help prevent and relieve many of the more uncomfortable symptoms of later pregnancy.

MONTH 7
WEEKS 28 TO 31

The seventh month of pregnancy is when many women who have more or less felt as if they weren't pregnant to this point really begin to feel what all those other people have been talking about. Heartburn, gassiness, indigestion, constipation, swollen legs and feet, spider veins, hemorrhoids—all of these lovelies can begin to arise as pregnancy weight accumulates and the belly continues to grow and press on surrounding structures.

I strongly believe that all these symptoms are worsened by eating a lot of animal products. Meats (which are almost completely devoid of fiber) will sit in your digestive system longer, causing increased heartburn, gas, constipation, and hemorrhoids. Also, consider this: When you are pregnant and consume dairy products, your body must process not only your own flood of estrogen, but also the hormones from the lactating cow or goat. Equal amounts of calcium and vitamin D can be found in most fortified organic almond, hemp, soy, or coconut milks. For these reasons (and others), if you are going to consume animal products, I encourage you to do so sparingly, and if possible, commit to choosing organically raised options.

Week by Week

WEEK 28 Your baby now weighs about 2½ pounds, and is kicking distinctly and forcefully. I actually started having dreams of wild ponies bucking and kicking when I was around 28 weeks pregnant with my youngest daughter. Funny enough, now she's four, and this is totally consistent with her little bad-ass personality. So if you have a strong kicker . . . take note.

Speaking of personality, your baby's brain development in the third trimester is tremendous. Nourish it with essential brain foods: omega-3 fatty acids, choline, and vitamin B_{12}.

How Big Is Baby?

WEEK 28	15 INCHES
WEEK 29	15½ INCHES
WEEK 30	15¾ INCHES
WEEK 31	16 INCHES
WEEK 31 WEIGHT	3⅓ POUNDS

WEEK 29 Baby is getting close to her ultimate birth length, and now is really starting to pack on the pounds by filling out with a layer of white fat cells that she can use to store energy. As this process progresses, her wrinkly and saggy excess skin begins to firm up and smooth out to that velvet we equate with the expression "soft as a baby's bottom." Your baby probably weighs just under 3 pounds now, and her movements are starting to calm down a bit as space inside becomes slightly more limited in proportion to her growing body.

Her skeleton is absorbing about 250 mg of calcium per day (this continues through the end of pregnancy), so make sure you are meeting your dietary calcium goals to ensure baby's strong bones.

WEEK 30 Your dreams may be extremely vivid during pregnancy. Fetal neurodevelopment experts consider it likely that your baby is dreaming as well! What could he possibly be dreaming about? Well, just as your dreams may be influenced by the sights and sounds and emotions that you experience throughout your day, the same may be true for your baby. So provide good material: laugh, sing, walk in nature, dance to your favorite jams, and be loving with your partner and yourself. Your physical and psychological health and well-being are likewise consequential to the good health and well-being of your baby.

What's on Your Plate?

More calcium, please! This, plus extra brain food (omega-3 fatty acids, choline, and vitamin B$_{12}$) are the elements to focus on. Ensure proper intake by trying your hand at these great recipes.

- BREAKFAST BURRITO (PAGE 100)
- CHOCOLATE CHIA PUDDING (PAGE 198)
- HIGH-PROTEIN OATMEAL (PAGE 108)
- OMEGA-3 SNACK MIX (PAGE 115)
- PERFECT ROASTED CHICKEN (PAGE 169)
- SPEEDY BROCCOLI AND CHEDDAR SOUP (PAGE 133)

WEEK 31 The fetal bone marrow has now taken over from the liver as the primary producer of red blood cells. This may sound somewhat technical, but just think of it as baby's time to fine-tune some very important functions as he prepares for his world debut! Your baby is also starting to build up his own vitamin and mineral stores, some of which he deposits in the new layer of white fat that is rapidly accumulating around his body. Your own fat accumulation should not be rapid, however, but slow and steady, aiming for that pound-per-week goal.

Swimming is a wonderful exercise that takes the weight off your tired feet, mobilizes and stretches out all your joints, and cools you down as you may begin to be prone to overheating. Swimming also offers you the rare opportunity to feel as light and nimble as a ballerina! To boot, it's a great way of getting a cardiovascular work-out without fear of falling or exacerbating back pain that can come from higher-impact activities. And here's a little secret: Generally speaking, the *more* you move, the *less* back pain you will have.

FAQ

I've been diagnosed with gestational diabetes. What diet plan will best control my blood sugar and keep my baby healthy and safe for the rest of the pregnancy and birth?

I strongly believe that a whole foods, plant-based diet is the best diet to both prevent *and reverse* insulin resistance and gestational diabetes (as well as Type 2 diabetes). Even if you received a diagnosis or have been prescribed oral glyce-mic control agents or insulin, it doesn't mean that you will have to take medication for the remainder of your pregnancy. You will need to check your blood sugar regularly, but try a little experiment (with the guidance of your OB doc-tor). I challenge you to try a vegan diet with no refined grains or added sugars (including neither calorie-containing nor non-nutritive sweeten-ers). Dairy in the form of milk or dairy products like cheese and yogurt are lesser known sources of sugars. Just try cutting them out and observe. I predict that your blood sugars will normalize almost immediately, and that within a week or two you will not require the medication. Taking a pill or an insulin injection may seem easier or save you from confronting food issues, but over the long term, it is not the healthiest way to live.

Calcium-Rich
FOODS

We need 1 gram per day of calcium, both during pregnancy and breastfeeding, as our bodies literally grow our baby's new bones and teeth. What we don't get in our diet will be taken out of our own calcium stores, so eat up! Twelve foods rich in calcium are:

	Bok choy		Kale
	Broccoli		Organic dairy or fortified nondairy milk (soy, almond, hemp, coconut)
	Broccoli rabe		Plain yogurt
	Collard greens		Sardines
	Edamame		Sesame seeds
	Figs		Tofu

MONTH 8
WEEKS 32 TO 35

Most women who choose to do so schedule their Demi Moore–style naked pregnancy photo session sometime during month 8. Rightly so, as you are very pregnant-looking at this point, but still have the energy and patience to do things like remember to schedule and pose for a pregnancy photo session. Regardless of your desires or inhibitions or self-image, give yourself a hug. You are a mother, and you are beautiful.

Your baby is still developing, but looks very much like the baby you will see in a few weeks. Most babies born prematurely in the eighth month of pregnancy survive, and many do quite well with the support of modern hospitals' neonatal intensive care units (NICUs). But continue to be patient; there are still important activities going on inside you. Baby is adding fat for insulation, and lung development is continuing.

How Big Is Baby?

WEEK 32	16¾ INCHES
WEEK 33	17 INCHES
WEEK 34	18 INCHES
WEEK 35	18 INCHES
WEEK 35 WEIGHT	5¼ POUNDS

Continue to eat full, nutrition-packed meals so you can keep your energy up and baby's body thriving. Some surprise uterine contractions may remind you that you are getting close to the end of your pregnancy, so while exercise is still important, be sure to take time to relax, reflect, and even journal about your amazing journey.

Week by Week

WEEK 32 Because the head is the heaviest part of the baby, most babies have done a little half-somersault and landed in the head-down vertex position by this week. Don't worry if this hasn't happened yet, because babies can still continue to turn spontaneously over the next few weeks, and some babies even turn at full term.

The fur-like lanugo that once covered your baby's entire body is beginning to shed, and more subcutaneous fat deposits continue to make her skin increasingly opaque.

WEEK 33 As your uterus continues to grow and stretch, more light is penetrating the amniotic sac. When your baby's eyes are open, his pupils now react to this light by dilating and constricting.

Your uterus is also starting to rev up its own activity, and you may begin to experience practice contractions known as Braxton-Hicks contractions, as your body prepares for delivery. These contractions feel like tightening that comes and goes at irregular intervals, and is not painful.

What's on Your Plate?

This month, zero in on fiber intake as well as vitamin C and choline. Make sure you get your probiotics to help ensure vaginal health for a good delivery. These delicious recipes will satisfy you and fill your collective nutritional needs.

- CHIA-BERRY SMOOTHIE (PAGE 103)
- OMEGA-3 SNACK MIX (PAGE 115)
- ZOODLES MARINARA (PAGE 182)
- WHEAT BERRY AND QUINOA BURGERS (PAGE 181)
- COD AND FENNEL STEW (PAGE 136)

WEEK 34 Your baby continues to gain weight at the rate of about ½ pound per week. If you experience an abrupt increase in your weight gain, bring it to your provider's attention; they will make sure you are within normal blood pressure readings and not spilling protein in your urine.

The vernix is increasing and thickening at this point. It's part of what makes a baby's skin so incredibly soft.

WEEK 35 By week 35, 97 percent of babies are positioned head-down in the womb. The volume of amniotic fluid, which peaked at about week 33, has now plateaued. At this point, there's less fluid in proportion to the volume of your growing baby, making further somersaults less likely, but not impossible.

These next few weeks really try to stay away from all added sugars and processed carbohydrates, which can compromise vaginal health. Eat immune-boosting foods like organic red bell peppers, organic strawberries, kiwis, and cooked shiitake, maitake, and crimini mushrooms. Eat fermented foods high in probiotics, as well as lots of good fiber-rich prebiotics. A healthy gut and vaginal flora in place helps prevent intra-uterine and neonatal infections. This also helps set up your baby's immune system to be healthy and robust for life.

FAQ

Can I eat flavored yogurt as my source of probiotics?
You can, but the impact in terms of probiotic benefits is minimal. Flavored yogurts are packed full of sugar and sweeteners and have very few actual live probiotic culture strains per serving. Instead, consider a good supplement—one containing at least 10 billion live organisms per serving (some blend of lactobacillus and bifidobacterium strains).

What about drinking flavored vitamin waters?
It's much more beneficial to drink pure filtered water stored in glass, or make your own flavored water by adding some sliced fruit. (see page 37). Prepared flavored waters are often sweetened with added sugars or artificial sweeteners and will trigger your cravings for sugary foods. However, if the choice is a vitamin water or a soda, by all means choose the former.

Iron-Rich

FOODS

The Institute of Medicine recommends 27 mg of iron per day in pregnancy, 9 mg a day while breastfeeding. Used in combination with foods high in vitamin C will dramatically increase the body's ability to absorb iron. Twelve foods rich in iron are:

	Black sesame seeds		Olives
	Dried apricots		Oysters
	Garbanzo beans		Spinach
	Kidney beans		Spirulina
	Lentils		Squash and pumpkin seeds
	Morel mushrooms		Swiss chard

MONTH 9
WEEKS 36 TO 41+

This is not just the home stretch; this is also the sexiest month of your pregnancy. I bet you didn't think that was coming. But think about it: You have the leading role in the most exclusively female undertaking there is. You are the goddess reclining and should be worshipped as such. Massages are fine at this point in pregnancy, so indulge, using organic, natural oils like vitamin E or olive or sesame oil. Don't skip the vulva and perineum—massage relaxes the tissues and makes them more pliant.

If you have access to a private pool or nudist beach and feel so inclined, swim naked. Having actual sex and orgasm at this point in the pregnancy can be very beneficial in terms of relaxing your hip flexors and allowing the baby's head to descend and engage in your pelvis. It can also promote cervical ripening and make labor easier. Best of all, sex does wonders for your sleep.

Speaking of sleep, try to bank up as much as you can this month. Epsom salt baths with lavender essential oil before bedtime will relax your mind and body; they also help prevent muscle spasms (especially in your back and legs).

Eat lightly and frequently, and focus on liquids. Soups, nutrient-rich smoothies, and fresh vegetable juices will give you the nutrition you need without making you feel overly full. And sigh, that overly full feeling is going to get more and more prominent until you feel like there is just not one more ounce of space within you, and about then, you will release.

Oh yes, it's time. You are going to birth your baby sometime in the next handful of weeks. And what a lucky baby, to be coming home with a healthy, vibrant, whole-foods-savvy mama like you.

Week by Week

WEEK 36 Keep up the immune-boosting fruits and veggies in small, frequent, light portions. Also, take a good probiotic supplement from now until the birth of your baby to optimize that birth canal. You can blend plant-based protein powders into your smoothies and kick up their nutrient punch with seed and nut butters. Puréed vegetable soups go down easily and won't give you that overstuffed feeling. And drink, drink, drink. Water is best.

How Big Is Baby?

WEEK 36	18½ INCHES
WEEK 37	19 INCHES
WEEK 38	19½ INCHES
WEEK 39	20 INCHES
WEEK 40	20 INCHES
WEEK 40 WEIGHT	7½ POUNDS

WEEK 37 At the completion of this gestational week (exactly 37 weeks from your LMP), your baby is officially considered full-term. That doesn't necessarily mean she is ready to be born. Some have not yet achieved fetal lung maturity to be able to breathe alone without support. The liver is still continuing to develop as well, and may not be fully prepared to process bilirubin (this is where the common issue of jaundice comes from) or regulate blood sugar levels.

In light of this, be patient—your body has a wonderful way of knowing the perfect time to release baby from your belly to your arms. Resist the urge to talk your provider into an elective induction of labor or C-section; let your body be delivery's guide. If you are maintaining a healthy diet and exercise regimen, chances are you are less likely to be experiencing side effects that might make you long for the pregnancy to end. Either way, just as you have been kind and gentle with your body throughout the pregnancy, try to extend this a few more weeks to give your baby the time it needs to finish prenatal growth.

WEEK 38 You may be "nesting" because your body knows it could go into labor at any time. You may have runs of contractions that come at regular intervals, or that feel much more intense than the Braxton-Hicks contractions you have been used to. This is completely normal and is all part of your body's amazing and methodical preparation for delivery. Stay hydrated with lots of fluids containing electrolytes (but not sugars). Real labor will declare itself as such and will come when the time is right.

WEEK 39 By the end of this week, your baby's lungs are very likely fully mature, and liver fully functional at processing bilirubin and regulating blood sugar levels. This was the week that I felt ready in all three of my pregnancies, and did everything in my human (but nonmedically intervening) power to help things along. This included walking 45 minutes on a treadmill at an 11 percent incline the night I went into labor with my first child. So much for patience, right?

WEEK 40 Even though the completion of this week ends with the all-powerful "due date" (a virtually meaningless mark on the calendar that rarely winds up being baby's birthday), it is also a week like any other week in your pregnancy. Take care of your body, sleep whenever you can, and sip healthy liquids as much as possible.

WEEKS 41–42 Ah, you've passed your due date. You may be ruffled by this fact, but it's really pretty common. That due date, in fact, is a pretty arbitrary date that (when obstetricians came up with the idea) simply represented statistically the midpoint by which time 50 percent of mothers will have delivered their babies. That means that 50 percent will not have delivered by 40 weeks.

Continue to practice all of your healthy, self-nurturing behaviors that you have learned

What's on Your Plate?

As the big day quickly approaches (or slowly, as you may feel), think about iron, vitamin B$_{12}$, probiotics, and water, which all play a role in helping you and baby get ready and feel good doing it! Drink lots of water, and if one day you can, let someone else do the cooking for you using some of the following recipes.

- DR. JENNIFER'S GREEN SMOOTHIE (PAGE 105)
- NO-COOK QUINOA PROTEIN BITES (PAGE 111)
- SPAGHETTI SQUASH PARMESAN (PAGE 184)
- COCONUT SOUP (PAGE 130)
- CREAMY MISO YOGURT DRESSING (PAGE 157)

over the course of your pregnancy. Your baby and your body will know when it's time to deliver.

Most important during these weeks, stay well hydrated and take advantage of any chance to rest. Once baby arrives, opportunities to nap may not come as easily!

FAQ

I've heard about some women eating their placenta after they deliver, and services that come and put it into capsules for you. Is this something I should consider?

Most mammals in nature (with the exception of marine mammals) eat their placentas. Humans, however, have a long tradition across many cultures of not eating it. Human placentophagy really only started gaining interest in the 1970s, and has now become something more discussed and practiced, particularly in the natural birthing community. As there is no double-blind randomized trial in the peer-reviewed literature to either support or refute the consuming of the placenta, I will say: do it (safely and hygienically) if you want to. It is a very protein- and iron-rich food, which also packs a ton of progesterone. If you choose to do it, I recommend one of the professional services that dehydrates, desiccates, and encapsulates the placenta so it can be taken back internally over time.

FOODS TO
Stimulate Breast Milk

With a baby coming shortly, you may want to start considering how to stimulate breast milk. The best thing you can do for your body is drink enough. Keep a glass of water by your side around the clock. Other foods can help, too. Top recommendations include:

Water
Keep it stored in glass. Add sliced fruit or herbs if you like. Mix water 1:1 with cactus, coconut, or maple sap waters for added minerals and electrolytes. Drink a giant glass of water every time you sit down to breast-feed.

Garlic
Researchers performed a study where they gave breast-feeding women garlic supplements. The babies of the women who received the garlic nursed longer, sucked harder, and drank more milk. This healing herb is also antibacterial, antiviral, and antifungal.

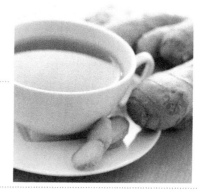

Raw vegetable juices
These have myriad benefits, among which are promoting healthy breast tissue and setting your baby up to accept vegetables later on.

Ginger
This lactogenic food promotes breast milk production, decreases nausea, helps digestion, clears respiratory symptoms, relieves stress, and strengthens immunity. Try ginger tea.

Carrots
Carrots are known to boost milk supply and improve later acceptance of carrots by infants.

Green (unripe) papaya
South Asian cultures use unripe papaya to help support breast-feeding mothers. This fruit has a relaxing property that helps with milk production.

Oatmeal
Oats are great for milk production. This anti-inflammatory complex carbohydrate also helps counter the constipation experienced by many breast-feeding women.

Fennel
Fennel contains a phytoestrogen that supports healthy breast tissue and lactation.

Nuts
Go for cashews, almonds, walnuts, and macadamia nuts, which are rich in omega-3s and nutrients that help support postpartum recovery and the breast-feeding process.

Sesame seeds
Sesame seeds—particularly black sesame—are believed to help increase milk supply. Sesame oil is also amazing in your hair and as a massage oil.

six

FOURTH TRIMESTER

You have given birth, either vaginally or by cesarean section, and are entering what we jokingly call the "fourth trimester." This is a special time for both mother and baby, where your baby exists outside of your body but is still intimately connected to you in so many ways. In fact, there's a saying: "The day your child is born is when your heart starts living outside your body."

Whether you breastfeed or not, the influence your own nutrition has on your baby is as important now as it was when you were connected by an umbilical cord and placenta. If you are breast-feeding, your baby will continue to capture the nutrients and tastes from everything you ingest. Like you, baby will react to certain foods better than others. If you are not breast-feeding, baby still needs you to be in top form to respond to his needs around the clock.

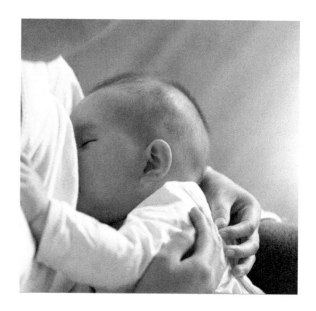

NUTRITION FOR BREAST-FEEDING MOTHERS

I'm not a pediatrician, so I'm not going to give you detailed advice on how to feed your baby. However, because of the overwhelming weight of scientific evidence, there is consensus that "breast is best." Exclusive breast-feeding is recommended for at least the first four months of life. That being said, for many reasons, many women cannot or do not choose to breast-feed. The caloric guideline of an extra 500 calories per day is for exclusive breast-feeders. If you are breast-feeding less often, you should consume less.

Okay, I lied. I'm going to make one plea for the pediatric diet. If you had a C-section or took antibiotics during your labor or delivery,

or your baby was given antibiotics after birth, add infant probiotic drops to your milk. If you are breast-feeding and have a pump, add these drops to the bottle of your pumped milk before feeding. Your baby's gut flora needs the support. High-quality science is increasingly recognizing how essential this is to human health.

Your baby will need to eat about every 2½ to 3½ hours, around the clock. To keep up with this, think of every breast-feeding session as an opportunity for you to drink a large 16-ounce serving of liquid with some electrolytes. Your colostrum comes out first, which is a scant, thick, highly nutrient-dense liquid, exceptionally rich in protective antibodies for your newborn. After a couple days, you will notice your milk supply increasing in volume and becoming less of a deep golden yellow and more of a yellow-white color.

Determined to lose my 30 pounds of baby weight, I hopped back on the treadmill three days after my first birth. Immediately, I saw a reduction in the volume of milk that I was able to produce. I realized that I needed to eat more carbohydrates and fats and exercise less in order to keep up with the 500 extra calories it took to produce all of that milk. So I changed my regimen. Without any exercise beyond light hiking, the pounds still melted off. And if you eat right, you will notice the same thing!

Good Nutrition During Breast-Feeding

Everything you put on, around, and inside your body can make it into your breast milk—everything from the mattress you sleep on, to the shampoo you use for your hair, to the foods and liquids you ingest every day. Do your best to choose healthy whole foods that will help your body recover from the birth and will fill your breast milk with important nutrients so baby can thrive. And just like your developing baby

What's on Your Plate?

It's as important as ever to eat well, especially if you're breast-feeding and even if you're not. Try to get extra protein, nutrient-rich calories (think avocados, nuts, seeds, raw nut butters), whole grains, and of course lots of water to stay hydrated. Here are some recipes that will keep Mama running the show like a pro.

- AVOCADO-HEMP SPREAD (PAGE 125)
- CRISPY OVEN FRIES (PAGE 154)
- EVERYDAY SPAGHETTI (PAGE 177)
- PEANUT BUTTER PROTEIN BARS (PAGE 116)
- POMEGRANATE GUACAMOLE (PAGE 122)
- VEGETABLE FRIED RICE (PAGE 180)

could taste the flavors of the foods you consumed in the amniotic fluid, she can taste flavors in your breast milk. You continue to shape your baby's taste palate and prepare her for a lifetime of healthy food choices. Almost universally, what's good for you is good for your baby, and what's not fabulous for you is not fabulous for your baby.

Passing It Along: How Not To

If you happen to consume something in the not-fabulous category, you can occasionally do what is known as "pump and dump" for various lengths of time after consumption. Different substances have different half-lives in the body. A half-life is the time it takes to metabolize or excrete half the quantity of the substance. Xanax is metabolized relatively quickly in the body, whereas Valium takes much longer. Yes, if you take these things and breast-feed, baby is taking them too. If possible, this is a good time to explore alternate remedies, such as meditation or aromatherapy.

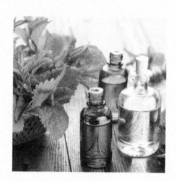

FAQ

Is there anything I can eat to help increase my breast milk supply?

We are so lucky to have all of human history as a virtual trial and error experiment to help answer this question that women have likely been asking since the beginning of our species. See page 87 for a list of "galactogogues," otherwise known as foods that increase milk supply. In addition to these, it is essential to stay well hydrated.

Is it OK to supplement my breast milk with formula?

Our brilliant bodies almost always make as much breast milk as our baby needs. Most women who begin with the idea that they are going to supplement, find they stop breastfeeding earlier. I recommend that you do at least the first 4 months with exclusive breast milk (direct from the breast and/or pumped and bottle-fed). It's most ideal for your baby's health and holds enormous benefits for your own.

Is it OK to drink alcohol while I'm breastfeeding?

If you consume alcohol, your breast milk will contain about the same level of alcohol as in your blood. You didn't drink in pregnancy because research shows alcohol consumption can have damaging effects to the development of your fetus. By this same logic, you'd be feeding alcohol to your growing newborn. Your child will have an opportunity try alcohol when he's 21, so let's keep early infancy as alcohol-and-drug-free as possible.

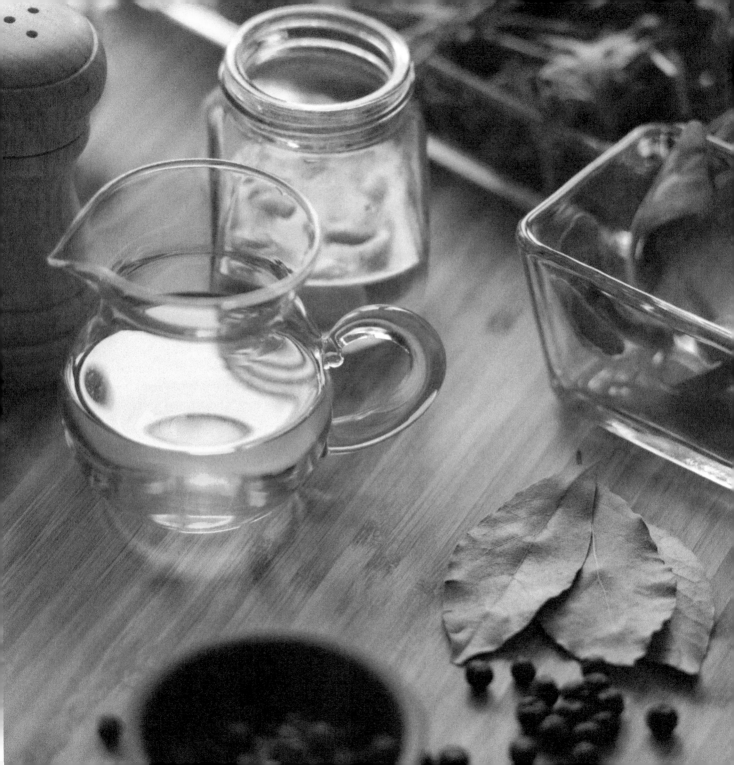

Part Three

RECIPES

It's time to get into the kitchen and put some of these healthy eating principles into practice. It might be intimidating at first, especially if you were not raised in a household that cooked. The good news is that when you cook with fresh, beautiful whole-food ingredients, it's pretty hard to mess it up. So find some groovy jams, kick off those shoes, and reclaim the cliché of literally being barefoot and pregnant in the kitchen!

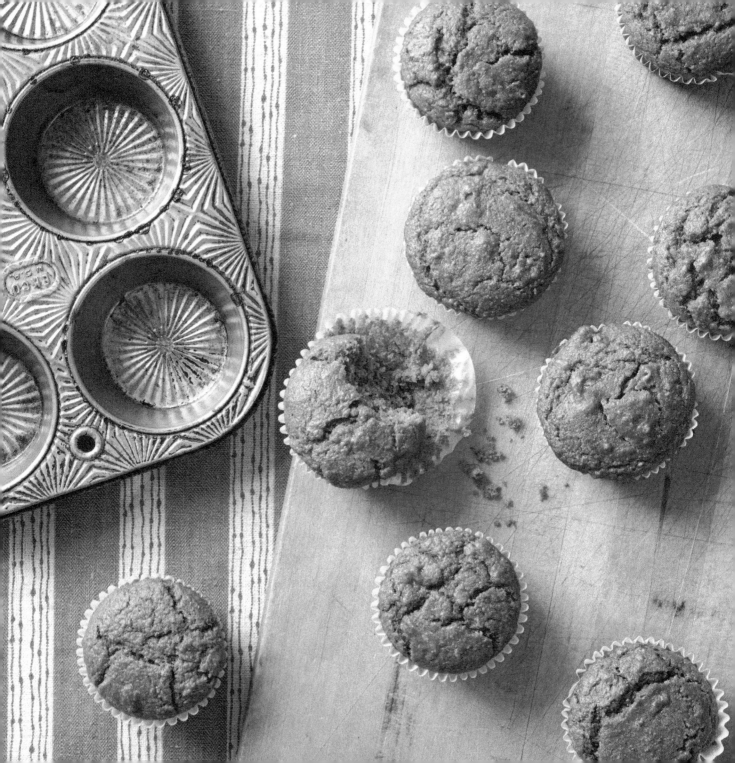

seven

BREAKFAST

AVOCADO TOAST

SERVES 1; PREP TIME: 5 MINUTES
COOK TIME: NONE

Sometimes the simplest recipes are the most delicious. This breakfast has it all, with minimal ingredients. Avocado's healthy fat and high-fiber whole-grain bread makes this an extra satisfying meal. Choose any variety of whole-grain bread, including gluten-free options like buckwheat and brown rice.

½ avocado, mashed

1 slice 100% whole-grain bread, toasted

Pinch coarse kosher salt

Freshly squeezed lemon juice

Spread the mashed avocado on the toast, season with salt, and sprinkle with fresh lemon juice to taste.

PER SERVING: Calories: 274; Total Fat 21g; Saturated Fat: 4g; Carbohydrates: 20g; Fiber: 9g; Protein: 6g

EGGS AND GREENS

SERVES 1; PREP TIME: 2 MINUTES
COOK TIME: 5 MINUTES

We should always make time for breakfast, even on mornings when you aren't feeling up to it. This recipe is filled with nutritious ingredients and is ready in minutes. Change out the mix-ins depending on your cravings. Any type of vegetable and even a sprinkle of cheese works well.

1 teaspoon olive oil

1 slice 100% whole-grain bread, torn into pieces

1 egg, beaten

½ cup baby spinach or chopped kale

Pinch kosher salt

Pinch freshly ground black pepper

1. Heat the olive oil in a small enameled skillet over medium heat.

2. Add the bread and toss to gently toast.

3. Add the egg and spinach. Season with salt and pepper.

4. Gently scramble the mixture until it is set, about 1 minute.

TIP: You can replace the egg in this recipe with protein-packed diced firm tofu.

PER SERVING: Calories: 176; Total Fat 10g; Saturated Fat: 2g; Carbohydrates: 15g; Fiber: 2g; Protein: 9g

WHOLE-GRAIN FRENCH TOAST

SERVES 4; PREP TIME: 5 MINUTES
COOK TIME:10 MINUTES

You may think of French toast only as a decadent treat, but it can actually be mighty healthy. The eggs and milk are the basis for an especially nutritious breakfast. Use fiber-rich whole-grain bread and top with lots of fresh fruit

2 large eggs

1 cup milk or almond milk

1 teaspoon pure vanilla extract

½ teaspoon ground cinnamon

4 teaspoons coconut oil

8 slices 100% whole-grain bread

Pure maple syrup

Fresh seasonal fruit, sliced

1. In a large bowl, whisk together the eggs, milk, vanilla, and cinnamon. Set aside.

2. Heat a large enameled skillet over medium heat. Add 1 teaspoon of the coconut oil.

3. Dip one slice of the bread into the milk mixture, soaking both sides well. Repeat for a second slice.

4. Place the two slices in the skillet and cook for 2 to 3 minutes on each side or until golden brown. Remove to a warmed plate.

5. Repeat with the remaining slices of bread, adding more coconut oil as needed.

6. Serve sprinkled with additional cinnamon, if desired. Top with maple syrup and fresh fruit.

PER SERVING (WITHOUT TOPPINGS): Calories: 247; Total Fat 10g; Saturated Fat: 6g; Carbohydrates: 26g; Fiber: 4g; Protein: 12g

RED AND GREEN FRITTATA

SERVES 2; PREP TIME: 10 MINUTES
COOK TIME: 10 MINUTES

Many healthy egg dishes choose egg whites as the star ingredient, but don't get rid of those yolks! This part of the egg is rich in antioxidants and omega-3 fats, plus there's just as much protein in the yolks as there is in the whites. Make this recipe for a crowd or for one and have some left-overs for lunch the next day.

4 large eggs, beaten

1 cup chopped green and red vegetables, such as spinach, bell pepper, tomato, and onion

2 tablespoons chopped fresh basil

¼ cup shredded part-skim mozzarella cheese, divided

⅛ teaspoon kosher salt

Freshly ground black pepper

1. Preheat the broiler.

2. Heat an ovenproof enameled skillet over medium heat.

3. In a large bowl, whisk the eggs. Stir in the vegetables, basil, and half of the cheese. Add the salt and season with pepper.

4. Pour the egg mixture into the skillet and gently scramble.

5. While the eggs are still runny, sprinkle with the remaining cheese and transfer to the oven.

6. Broil for 1 to 2 minutes, watching carefully, or until the eggs are set and the cheese is melted.

TIP: Use any combination of vegetables and cheese. The eggs are a blank canvas.

PER SERVING: Calories: 193; Total Fat 13g; Saturated Fat: 5g; Carbohydrates: 3g; Fiber: 1g; Protein: 17g

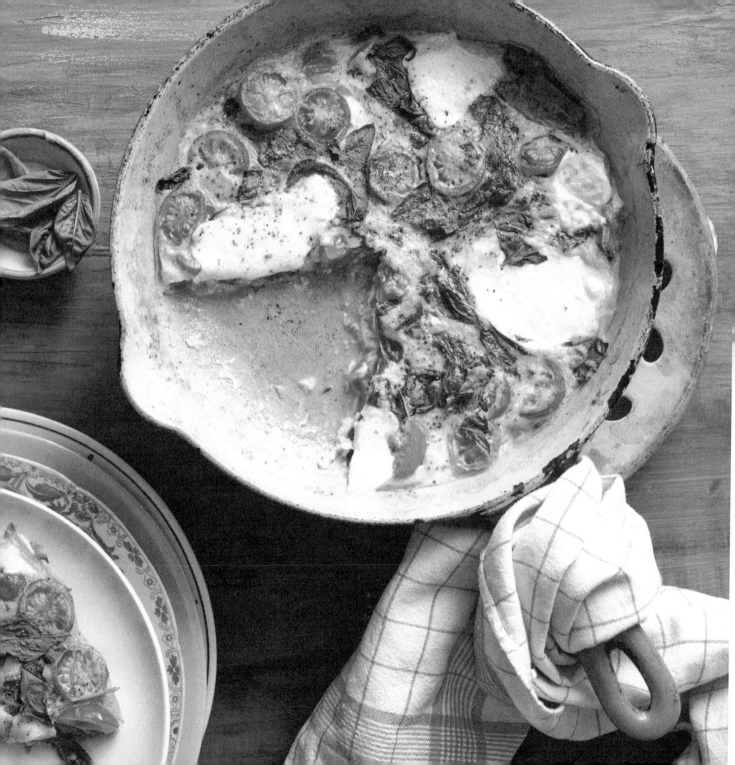

BREAKFAST BURRITO

SERVES 1; PREP TIME: 5 MINUTES
COOK TIME: 5 MINUTES

This burrito will keep you satisfied all morning long. Whipping it up for breakfast will help get in servings of whole grains and veggies right at the start of your day. Instead of cheese, avocado makes this wrap extra special.

1 large egg

1 egg white

Pinch kosher salt

Pinch freshly ground black pepper

1 medium whole-grain tortilla, warmed

¼ cup diced tomato

¼ cup diced avocado

Hot sauce for serving (optional)

1. Heat an enameled skillet over medium heat.

2. In a small bowl, whisk the egg and egg white until well beaten. Season with salt and pepper.

3. Add the egg mixture to the pan and gently scramble until the eggs are set.

4. Place the warmed tortilla on a serving plate, and put the eggs in the center of the tortilla. Top with the tomato, avocado, and hot sauce, if using.

5. Roll up the tortilla and serve.

TIP: Try a gluten-free tortilla made from corn, brown rice, or buckwheat.

PER SERVING: Calories: 282; Total Fat 13g; Saturated Fat: 3g; Carbohydrates: 28g; Fiber: 6g; Protein: 14g

KALE OMELET

SERVES 1; PREP TIME: 5 MINUTES
COOK TIME: 5 MINUTES

This dish offers another great way to get your greens. Kale is filled with insoluble fiber that helps eliminate constipation. This is a great recipe to try if you don't think you like kale. When gently sautéed it becomes slightly sweet, nutty, and delicious. If you're looking for a dairy-free option, omit the Swiss cheese or replace it with a vegan version.

1 egg

2 egg whites

1 tablespoon water

Kosher salt

Freshly ground black pepper

1 cup chopped kale

1 ounce lowfat Swiss cheese, grated

1. Heat an enameled skillet over medium heat.

2. In a medium bowl, add the egg, egg whites, and water. Season with salt and pepper, and whisk.

3. Add the kale to the egg mixture.

4. Pour the egg mixture into the skillet and cook for 1 to 2 minutes or until the eggs begin to set. Using a spatula, gently pull in the sides of the omelet to let the uncooked egg run to the edge of the pan.

5. Put the cheese on half of the omelet and gently fold the omelet over. Cook for 2 minutes or until the cheese is melted.

TIP: Try this omelet for lunch with added flavor from roasted red peppers.

PER SERVING: Calories: 218; Total Fat 10g; Saturated Fat: 5g; Carbohydrates: 9g; Fiber: 3g; Protein: 21g

EGG AND KALE STACKERS

SERVES 1; PREP TIME: 5 MINUTES
COOK TIME: 10 MINUTES

Undercooked eggs can be a food safety hazard, so this version of "Eggs Benedict" uses eggs that are cooked through. You can also use scrambled eggs if you prefer.

1 whole-wheat English muffin, split

1 teaspoon olive oil

2 eggs

1 cup steamed kale or Swiss chard

4 thin slices avocado

1. Toast the English muffin.

2. Heat 1 teaspoon of olive oil in a skillet, heat, and break the eggs into the skillet. Fry until the yolks are no longer runny.

3. To assemble, on each muffin half put the kale on 2 slices of avocado, and top with a fried egg.

TIP: Food safety is important for pregnant women because they have a compromised immune system. Make sure all meat, eggs, and fish are cooked to the proper internal temperature.

PER SERVING: Calories: 452; Total Fat 24g; Saturated Fat: 6g; Carbohydrates: 42g; Fiber: 9g; Protein: 20g

TOFU SCRAMBLE

SERVES 1; PREP TIME: 5 MINUTES
COOK TIME: 10 MINUTES

Tofu is a wonderful way to get in a serving of protein for breakfast. Tofu takes on the flavor of the vegetables and adds hunger-fighting protein to the mix. Tofu also provides calcium, a bone-building mineral that most women don't get enough of.

2 teaspoons olive oil

1 cup chopped vegetables, like onion, peppers, and mushrooms

¾ cup firm tofu, diced

Kosher salt

Freshly ground black pepper

1 teaspoon chopped fresh chives

1. Heat the oil in a small skillet over medium heat.

2. Add the vegetables and sauté until tender.

3. Add the tofu, season with salt and pepper, and sauté until tofu is heated through.

4. Serve hot, garnished with the chives.

PER SERVING: Calories: 274; Total Fat 18g; Saturated Fat: 3g; Carbohydrates: 16g; Fiber: 6g; Protein: 19g

CHIA-BERRY SMOOTHIE

**SERVES 1; PREP TIME: 5 MINUTES
COOK TIME: NONE**

Chia seeds add a daily dose of omega-3 fats, and coconut water is loaded with potassium for a healthy heart. Freeze the yogurt, berries, chia seeds, and banana ahead of time in a reseal-able bag. On busy mornings just toss the frozen ingredients in the blender along with the coco-nut water.

½ cup lowfat vanilla yogurt

1 cup berries, frozen

1 tablespoon chia seeds

½ banana, sliced

½ cup coconut water

Combine yogurt, berries, chia seeds, banana, and coconut water in a blender. Blend until smooth and serve in a tall glass.

PER SERVING: Calories: 295; Total Fat 6g; Saturated Fat: 2g; Carbohydrates: 55g; Fiber: 11g; Protein: 10g

BANANA-WALNUT SMOOTHIE BOWL

**SERVES 1; PREP TIME: 5 MINUTES
COOK TIME: NONE**

It's oddly satisfying to eat your smoothie with a spoon, and a smoothie is a lot healthier than ice cream. Forget about added sugar. This smoothie is naturally sweetened with dates. Walnuts—rich in omega-3 fats—give this breakfast just the hint of crunchy goodness it needs.

2 ripe bananas

1 dates, pitted and roughly chopped

¼ cup walnuts

½ cup lowfat milk or almond milk

Ice

Walnuts, chia seeds, pepitas (shelled pumpkin seeds), or chopped fruit, for topping

1. Place bananas, dates, walnuts, milk, and ice in a blender. Blend until smooth.

2. Pour into bowls and add the desired top-pings. Dig in.

TIP: There are so many nondairy milk alterna-tives to choose from, and they all have different flavors and nutrients to offer. Experiment with options made from hemp, almond, cashew, rice, and coconut to see which is your favorite.

PER SERVING (WITHOUT TOPPINGS): Calories: 497; Total Fat 21g; Saturated Fat: 3g; Carbohydrates: 75g; Fiber: 9g; Protein: 12g

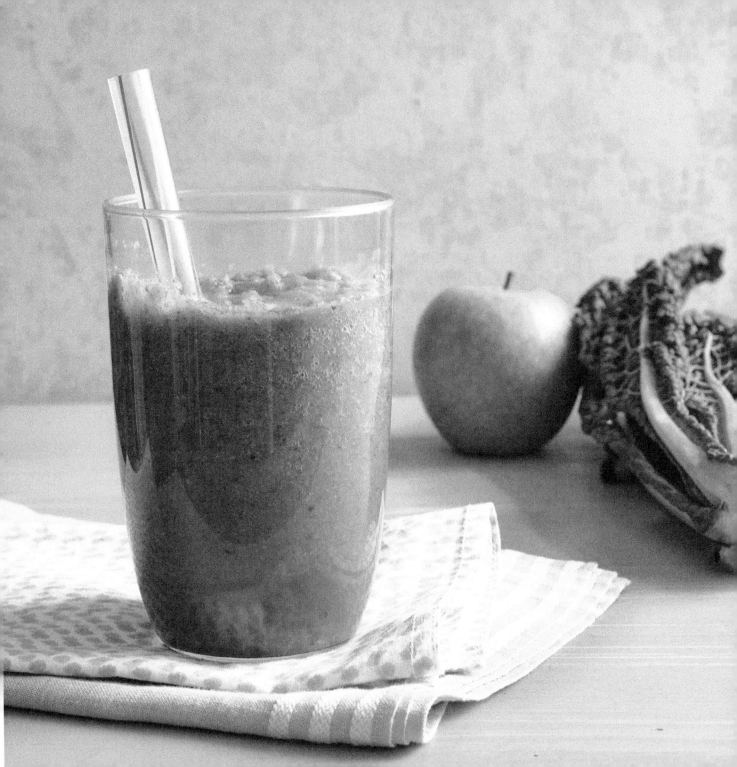

DR. JENNIFER'S GREEN SMOOTHIE

SERVES 1; PREP TIME: 5 MINUTES
COOK TIME: NONE

This smoothie is a great starter if you want to get into making your own green drinks. Filled with vitamin-rich greens and a hint of fresh ginger to curb nausea, it tastes absolutely amazing.

1 cup water

½ cucumber, chopped

½ cup chopped kale

1 cup baby spinach

1 green apple, cored and quartered

Juice of 1 freshly squeezed lemon

1-inch piece peeled chopped fresh ginger

Ice

Place the water, cucumber, kale, spinach, apple, lemon juice, ginger, and ice in a blender. Blend until smooth and serve in a tall glass.

TIP: Be sure to add the water first to make the smoothie easier to blend.

PER SERVING: Calories: 154; Total Fat 1g; Saturated Fat: 0g; Carbohydrates: 37g; Fiber: 6g; Protein: 4g

MANGO-BANANA SMOOTHIE

SERVES 1; PREP TIME: 5 MINUTES
COOK TIME: NONE

A good smoothie is about balance. Combine frozen fruit with protein-packed Greek yogurt and a splash of water, and you have all your breakfast bases covered. Potassium-packed banana is a perfect ingredient for a super creamy drink.

½ medium sliced banana, frozen

½ cup peeled mango chunks, frozen

4 ounces nonfat Greek yogurt

Water

Place the banana, mango, yogurt, and water in a blender. Blend until smooth, adding just enough water to get the desired consistency.

TIP: Cut down on wasted foods. When bananas are about to go bad on the counter, transfer them to a resealable freezer bag and freeze.

PER SERVING: Calories: 214; Total Fat 1g; Saturated Fat: 0g; Carbohydrates: 45g; Fiber: 3g; Protein: 7g

APPLE PIE OATMEAL

SERVES 1; PREP TIME: 5 MINUTES
COOK TIME: 10 MINUTES

If you're craving apple pie, you're in luck with this healthy, easy, and delicious way to kick off your day! Substitute milk with almond or coconut milk for a dairy-free alternative.

1 cup lowfat milk or nondairy milk alternative

Pinch kosher salt

1 cinnamon stick

½ cup rolled oats

½ cup diced apples

2 tablespoons chopped almonds

1. Place the milk, salt, and cinnamon stick in a saucepan, and bring to a simmer over medium-high heat.

2. Stir in the oats and apples.

3. Reduce the heat to medium-low and cook for 5 to 7 minutes, stirring frequently.

4. Serve hot, topped with the almonds.

PER SERVING: Calories: 363; Total Fat 11g; Saturated Fat: 2g; Carbohydrates: 52g; Fiber: 7g; Protein: 9g

REFRIGERATOR OATS

SERVES 1; PREP TIME: 10 MINUTES, PLUS
OVERNIGHT; COOK TIME: NONE

What's not to love about a make-ahead breakfast? This dish is filled with important nutrients like soluble fiber, calcium, and omega-3 fats, and it requires absolutely no effort at breakfast time, other than digging in.

½ cup rolled oats

2 teaspoons chia seeds

¼ teaspoon chopped fresh orange zest

1 cup vanilla almond milk

Fresh fruit and chopped nuts, for serving

1. Combine the oats, chia seeds, orange zest, and almond milk in a jar and stir to combine.

2. Cover and store in the refrigerator overnight.

3. Serve, topped with fresh fruit and chopped nuts.

PER SERVING (WITHOUT FRESH FRUIT): Calories: 209; Total Fat: 7g; Saturated Fat: 1g; Carbohydrates: 28g; Fiber: 7g; Protein: 7g

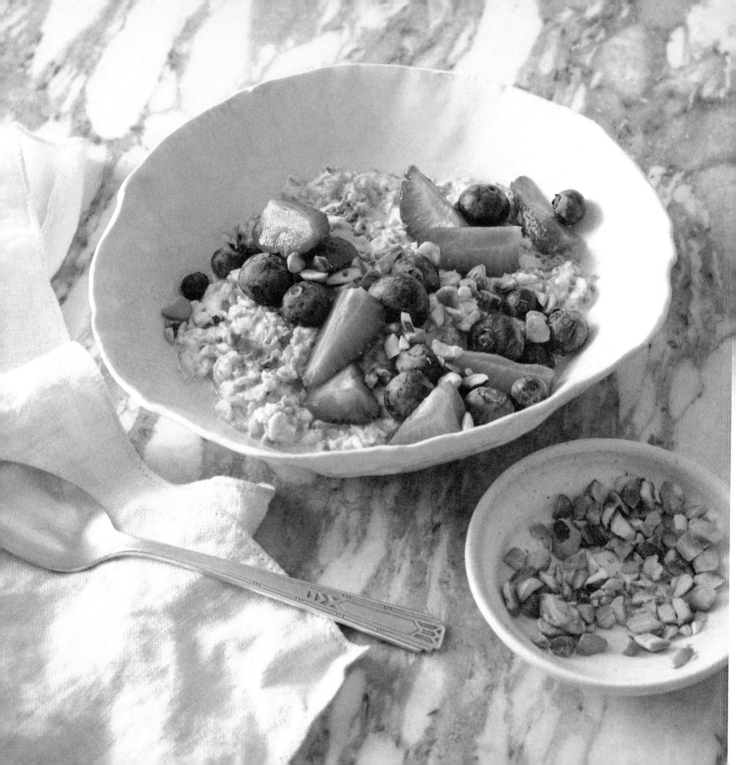

HIGH-PROTEIN OATMEAL

SERVES 2; PREP TIME: 5 MINUTES
COOK TIME: 10 MINUTES

Greek yogurt and milk give this oatmeal amazing texture, creamy flavor, and lots of hunger-fighting protein. Oats are high in soluble fiber, which aids digestion and supports heart health. For another whole-grain option, make this dish with buckwheat cereal or leftover quinoa.

1 cup rolled oats

Pinch kosher salt

2 cups skim milk

1 cup 2% plain Greek yogurt

Fresh berries, for topping

1. In a medium saucepan over medium-high heat, combine the oats, salt, and milk.

2. Bring to a simmer, reduce the heat to low, and cook for 5 minutes, stirring frequently until thick and creamy.

3. Add the yogurt and stir in. Serve topped with berries.

PER SERVING (WITHOUT TOPPING): Calories: 496; Total Fat: 8g; Saturated Fat: 4g; Carbohydrates: 71g; Fiber: 8g; Protein: 27g

STEEL-CUT OVERNIGHT OATS

SERVES 4; PREP TIME: 5 MINUTES
COOK TIME: OVERNIGHT

Mix up this oatmeal in the slow cooker the night before and wake up to a hot breakfast. Steel-cut oats have a heartier texture than traditional rolled oats, with a pleasantly chewy texture and nutty flavor. They can take longer to cook on the stove, so this slow cooker method is especially handy.

1 cup steel-cut oats

4 cups water

¼ teaspoon kosher salt

1 cup dried fruit, like raisins, cranberries, or apricots

Pure maple syrup, for serving (optional)

1. Combine the oats, water, salt, and dried fruit in a slow cooker and stir.

2. Set to low and cook for 8 hours.

3. Serve topped with a drizzle of maple syrup, if desired.

PER SERVING: Calories: 278; Total Fat: 3g; Saturated Fat: 1g; Carbohydrates: 53g; Fiber: 6g; Protein: 7g

VEGAN BANANA MUFFINS

MAKES 16 MUFFINS; PREP TIME: 15 MINUTES
COOK TIME: 20 MINUTES

These muffins are free of dairy and eggs, but you won't even miss them. Bananas keep them extra moist, and natural sweeteners like maple syrup impart a wonderful flavor. Make plenty and store leftovers in the freezer. For a special treat, mix in some cacao nibs or vegan chocolate chips.

½ cup pure maple syrup

2 ripe bananas, mashed

1 teaspoon ground cinnamon

¼ cup coconut oil

1 teaspoon pure vanilla extract

1 cup unsweetened soy milk

2 cups whole-wheat pastry flour

1 tablespoon ground flaxseed

2 teaspoon baking soda

½ teaspoon kosher salt

1. Preheat the oven to 350°F.

2. Line two 8-cup standard muffin tins with paper muffin cups.

3. In a large bowl, combine the maple syrup, bananas, cinnamon, coconut oil, vanilla, and soy milk. Whisk well to combine.

4. In a large bowl, sift the pastry flour, flaxseed, baking soda, and salt, and whisk gently to combine.

5. Add the syrup mixture to the flour mixture and stir together to make a batter.

6. Using a ⅓-cup measuring cup, scoop the batter into the prepared muffin tins.

7. Bake for 20 to 25 minutes or until a toothpick poked into the center of a muffin comes out clean.

PER MUFFIN: Calories: 135; Total Fat: 4g; Saturated Fat: 0g; Carbohydrates: 22g; Fiber: 2g; Protein: 3g

RAISIN FLAXSEED GRANOLA

MAKES 4 CUPS; PREP TIME: 5 MINUTES
COOK TIME: 10 MINUTES

Homemade granola is tastier and healthier than anything out of a box. To keep this recipe gluten-free, use certified gluten-free rolled oats.

Olive oil, for greasing pan

2 cups rolled oats

2 tablespoons flaxseed

2 tablespoons shelled sunflower seeds

½ cup shredded unsweetened coconut

¼ teaspoon kosher salt

¼ cup honey

2 tablespoons coconut oil

1 cup raisins

1. Preheat the oven to 300°F.

2. Grease a large baking sheet with olive oil.

3. In a large bowl, combine the oats, flaxseed, sunflower seeds, coconut, salt, honey, and coconut oil.

4. Pour the mixture onto the baking sheet and smooth out evenly. Bake, stirring occasionally, until golden brown, about 10 minutes.

5. When the mixture is cool, stir in the raisins.

6. Store in an airtight container at room temperature for up to 2 weeks.

PER SERVING (¼ CUP): Calories: 112; Total Fat: 5g; Saturated Fat: 2g; Carbohydrates: 21g; Fiber: 2g; Protein: 2g

GREEK YOGURT PARFAIT

SERVES 1; PREP TIME: 5 MINUTES
COOK TIME: NONE

Greek yogurt is higher in protein than traditional yogurts, and it's lower in lactose so it can be tolerated better by folks with issues digesting dairy. As an additional healthy attribute this yogurt is filled with tummy-pleasing probiotics to help calm the digestive system.

1 cup plain nonfat Greek yogurt

1 tablespoon dried unsweetened coconut chips

¼ cup granola or whole-grain cereal

1 cup chopped fresh fruit

Honey

1. Layer in a serving glass, alternating the yogurt, coconut chips, granola, and fruit.

2. Drizzle with the honey and serve.

TIP: Try a cultured nondairy yogurt made from almond milk. They come in a variety of flavors and have wonderful texture.

PER SERVING: Calories: 347; Total Fat: 6g, Saturated Fat: 4g, Carbohydrate: 49g, Protein: 22g, Fiber: 9g

NO-COOK QUINOA PROTEIN BITES

MAKES 12 BITES; PREP TIME: 15 MINUTES
COOK TIME: NONE

Eating protein at every meal is important to help meet the increased metabolic demands of pregnancy. These bite-size power snacks are perfect for a quick breakfast before work or after a morning workout. When you're craving chocolate, toss in a few mini chocolate chips.

½ cup dry quinoa

¼ cup raw almond butter

½ cup rolled oats

2 large pitted dates, finely chopped

¼ cup chopped nuts

¼ cup mixed seeds, like sunflower, chia, and flax

Kosher salt

1. Pulse dry quinoa in a food processor or high-speed blender until it makes a fine flour.

2. In a medium bowl, add the quinoa flour and combine with the almond butter, oats, dates, nuts, and mixed seeds, stirring well to combine.

3. Using a tablespoon or small ice cream scoop, form the quinoa mixture into 12 small balls.

4. Store in an airtight container in the refrigerator for up to 1 week.

PER BITE: Calories: 104; Total Fat: 6g; Saturated Fat: 1g; Carbohydrates: 11g; Fiber: 2g; Protein: 3g

VEGETABLE CREAM CHEESE

MAKES 16 SERVINGS; PREP TIME: 10 MINUTES
COOK TIME: NONE

Make a batch of this veggie-filled spread for whole-grain toast, sandwiches, or for dipping stalks of celery—it's addictive! Many store-bought versions are low in veggies, but this one is jam-packed full of veggies.

8 ounces lowfat cream cheese, at room temperature

2 tablespoons finely chopped carrot

2 tablespoons finely chopped radish

2 tablespoons finely chopped scallions

1 tablespoon chopped fresh dill

¼ teaspoon kosher salt

Freshly ground black pepper

Combine all ingredients in a small bowl and mix well. Store in an airtight container in the refrigerator for up to 1 week.

TIP: Try this same method to make a veggie-spiked hummus.

PER TABLESPOON: Calories: 51; Total Fat 2g; Saturated Fat: 1g; Carbohydrates: 1g; Fiber: 0g; Protein: 1g

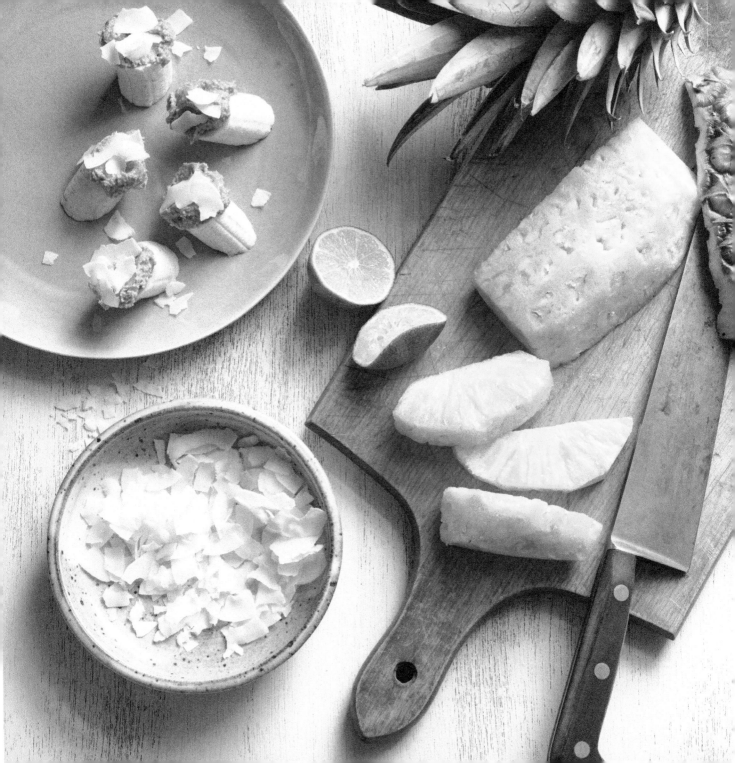

eight

SNACKS

···

CRUNCHY CURRY CHICKPEAS

MAKES 6 SERVINGS; PREP TIME: 5 MINUTES
COOK TIME: 40 MINUTES

Some pregnant women can't get enough spice and these crunchy bean snacks are way more satisfying than greasy chips. The turmeric in curry powder is a potent antioxidant to help protect cells and fight inflammation. If you and spice aren't getting along during your pregnancy, these snacks are still delicious made with just olive oil and salt.

1 (15-ounce) can chickpeas, drained and rinsed

1 tablespoon extra-virgin olive oil

½ teaspoon sea salt, plus more for sprinkling

1 teaspoon curry powder

1. Preheat the oven to 350°F.

2. Drain the chickpeas and dry well with a paper towel. Place on a baking sheet.

3. In a small bowl, combine the olive oil, salt, and curry powder. Pour over the chickpeas and stir together to coat well.

4. Bake for 40 to 50 minutes, turning periodically, until crisp and sizzling.

5. Sprinkle with sea salt.

TIP: Once cooled, store the chickpeas in an airtight container at room temperature for up to 1 week.

TIP: Instead of buying canned chickpeas, look for tetra-packed varieties so there's no concern about bisphenol A- (or BPA-) lined cans.

PER SERVING (¼ CUP): Calories: 159; Total Fat: 5g; Saturated Fat: 0g; Carbohydrates: 23g; Fiber: 7g; Protein: 7g

OMEGA-3 SNACK MIX

**MAKES 14 SERVINGS; PREP TIME: 5 MINUTES
COOK TIME: NONE**

Omega-3 fatty acids are vital for proper neurological development for a growing baby, and they also help keep mom's heart and skin healthy. Divide this snack mix into individual servings in a small resealable bag and toss in your tote for a healthy snack at the office and on the go.

1 cup walnuts

½ cup raisins

1 cup dried soy nuts

1 cup flaxseed granola

1. In a medium bowl, combine the walnuts, raisins, soy nuts, and granola and toss to combine.

2. Store in an airtight container at room temperature for up to 2 weeks.

PER SERVING (¼ CUP): Calories: 121; Total Fat: 9g; Saturated Fat: 1g; Carbohydrates: 14g; Fiber: 1g; Protein: 4g

CHOCOLATE CRUNCH MIX

**MAKES 16 SERVINGS; PREP TIME: 5 MINUTES
COOK TIME: NONE**

This snack mix is the answer to all those sweet, salty, and chocolate cravings, and you can feel good about eating it. Make the full recipe and store in an airtight container. To portion out, use a ¼-cup measure as a scoop so you get the proper amount every time.

1 cup cacao nibs or dark chocolate chips

1 cup slivered almonds

2 cups quinoa crisps (see Tip)

1. In a medium bowl, add the cacao nibs, almonds, and quinoa crisps and toss to combine.

2. Store in an airtight container at room temperature for up to 2 weeks.

TIP: You can find quinoa crisps at some health food stores or online, but you can also make your own. Toast precooked quinoa with a pinch of sea salt on a baking sheet in a 350°F oven for 10 to 15 minutes until crisp.

PER SERVING (¼ CUP): Calories: 112; Total Fat: 8g; Saturated Fat: 2g; Carbohydrates: 9g; Fiber: 4g; Protein: 4g

PEANUT BUTTER PROTEIN BARS

MAKES 12 BARS; PREP TIME: 10 MINUTES
COOK TIME: 20 MINUTES

Can't get enough peanut butter? These bars make a healthy and satisfying snack any time of day. These are a great bedtime snack because they are filled with protein and fiber. These will give you some of those extra calories you need to help sustain a healthy pregnancy in the second and third trimesters.

Olive oil, for coating the baking dish

¼ cup pure maple syrup

½ cup natural peanut butter

½ cup unsweetened almond or coconut milk

¼ cup vanilla protein powder

1 tablespoon coconut oil

1 teaspoon pure vanilla extract

1 cup rolled oats

2 cups puffed brown rice

½ cup chopped peanuts

½ cup dried banana chips, roughly chopped

½ cup pepitas (shelled pumpkin seeds)

½ teaspoon kosher salt

1. Coat a 9-by-9-inch baking dish with olive oil and set aside.

2. Preheat the oven to 325°F.

3. In a small saucepan, combine the maple syrup, peanut butter, almond milk, protein powder, coconut oil, and vanilla.

4. Stir together and cook over medium-low just until the mixture begins to bubble, 2 to 3 minutes.

5. In a large bowl, combine the oats, puffed rice, peanuts, banana chips, pepitas, and salt. Toss well.

6. Pour the warm peanut butter mixture over the oatmeal mixture and stir with a spatula until combined.

7. Transfer to the prepared baking dish and spread out evenly, pressing firmly.

8. Bake 15 minutes. Remove from the oven, let cool completely, and cut into 12 bars.

9. Store in an airtight container at room temperature for up to 1 week.

TIP: Be sure to buy natural peanut butter instead of those spiked with sugar and added oils. The only ingredients should be peanuts and salt.

PER BAR: Calories: 214; Total Fat: 14g; Saturated Fat: 4g; Carbohydrates: 18g; Fiber: 3g; Protein: 9g

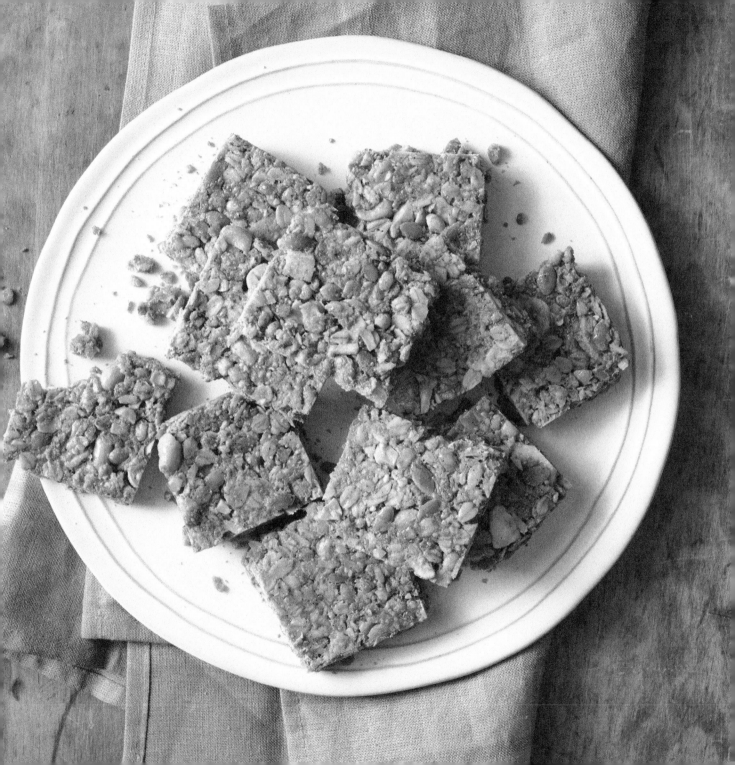

PEACH CHIA BREAKFAST PUDDING

SERVES 4; PREP TIME: 5 MINUTES,
PLUS 4 HOURS TO OVERNIGHT TO CHILL
COOK TIME: NONE

Use chia seeds rich in omega-3s to make this decadent velvety pudding without all the fat and calories. If peaches aren't in season, you can often find them in the frozen fruit section of your market. Otherwise, use any fresh seasonal fruit.

2 cups unsweetened soy or coconut milk

½ cup white chia seeds

1 cup chopped fresh peaches

1. In a large bowl, add the soy milk and chia seeds and whisk to combine.

2. Cover and place in the refrigerator to set for at least 4 hours or overnight.

3. Serve topped with the chopped peaches.

TIP: To keep chia seeds fresh, store in an airtight container in a cool, dry place.

PER SERVING: Calories: 212; Total Fat: 11g; Saturated Fat: 1g; Carbohydrates: 23g; Fiber: 12g; Protein: 6g

TROPICAL FRUIT SALAD

SERVES 6; PREP TIME: 10 MINUTES
COOK TIME: NONE

Keeping cut-up fruit on hand in the fridge gives you healthy choices when peering into the refrigerator. The sweet, juicy, and tangy fruit helps keep you hydrated and quells sugar cravings. For a special treat, serve with a dollop of lowfat plain yogurt.

2 kiwis, peeled

2 mangos, peeled

1 small pineapple, peeled and cored

2 large bananas, peeled

Juice of 1 lime

1. Cut the kiwis, mangos, pineapple, and bananas into large chunks, and put them in a large bowl. Add the lime juice and toss to coat.

2. Store in an airtight container in the refrigerator for up to 2 days.

PER SERVING: Calories: 152; Total Fat: 1g; Saturated Fat: 0g; Carbohydrates: 39g; Fiber: 5g; Protein: 2g

STRAWBERRY FRUIT LEATHER

MAKES 12 FRUIT LEATHERS;
PREP TIME: 10 MINUTES
COOK TIME: 3 HOURS 15 MINUTES,
PLUS OVERNIGHT

Pass on kiddie treats that are made from highly processed ingredients and no real fruit. This homemade fruit leather recipe is well worth the time it takes to make it. Your little ones will love having this treat in their lunchboxes.

2 cups chopped hulled fresh strawberries

2 tablespoons honey

1. Preheat the oven to 170°F. Line a baking sheet with a silicone baking mat and set aside.

2. In a medium saucepan, bring the strawberries and honey to a boil over medium-high heat and cook, stirring often, for about 5 minutes. Pureé using an immersion blender, countertop blender, or food processor.

3. Cook over medium-high heat, stirring frequently, for 10 to 15 minutes or until thick and syrupy.

4. Pour the hot fruit mixture onto the prepared baking sheet and spread evenly into a rectangle.

5. Bake for 3 hours, then turn off the oven and allow to sit in the oven overnight.

6. Cut into strips with a pizza cutter and roll each strip in a piece of parchment paper. Store the fruit leather rolls in an airtight container at room temperature for up to 1 week.

PER FRUIT LEATHER: Calories: 19; Total Fat: 0g; Saturated Fat: 0g; Carbohydrates: 5g; Fiber: 1g; Protein: 0g

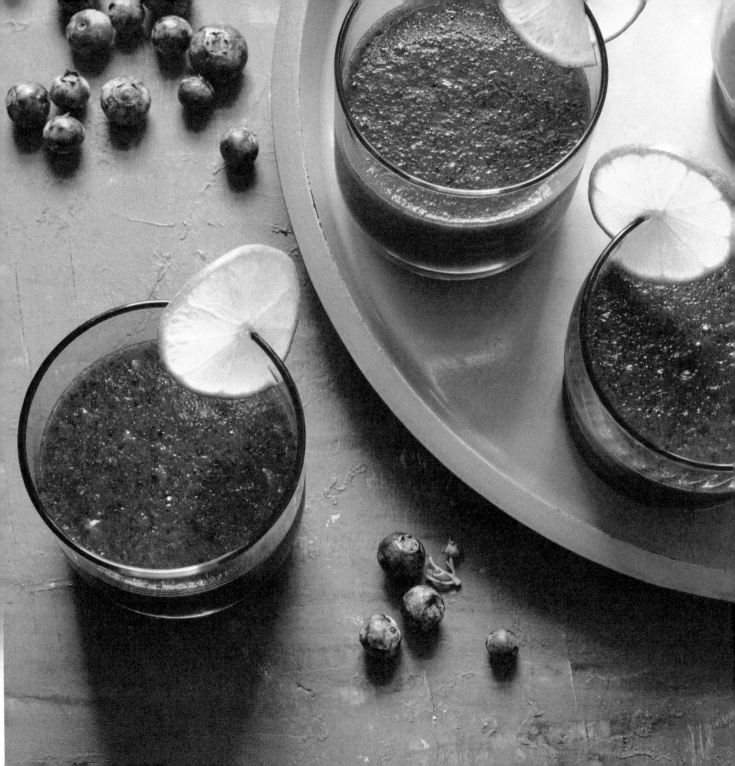

WILD WATERMELON COOLER

SERVES 1; PREP TIME: 5 MINUTES
COOK TIME: NONE

Enjoy this cooler when you need a boost of hydration and refreshment, or when you're dying for a cocktail. Frozen wild blueberries are higher in antioxidants than traditional blueberries and are packed at the peak of freshness. You will find them in the freezer section year-round.

1 cup cubed watermelon

1 cup frozen wild blueberries

½ cup water

Juice of ½ lime

1. In the blender, add the watermelon, berries, water, and lime juice.

2. Blend until smooth and serve in a tall glass.

PER SERVING: Calories: 149; Total Fat: 1g; Saturated Fat: 0g; Carbohydrates: 32g; Fiber: 5g; Protein: 3g

BASIL HUMMUS

MAKES 12 SERVINGS; PREP TIME: 10 MINUTES
COOK TIME: NONE

Homemade hummus is easy to make and is packed with nutrients, including fiber, iron, protein, and heart-healthy fats. Tahini is a paste made from sesame seeds. It's high in healthy unsaturated fats and gives hummus its nutty flavor.

2 (15-ounce) cans chickpeas

3 tablespoons sesame tahini

¼ cup extra-virgin olive oil

Juice of ½ lemon

½ cup fresh basil leaves

¼ teaspoon kosher salt

Freshly ground black pepper

Baby carrots, celery sticks, sliced cucumber, and pita chips, for serving

1. Rinse and drain the chickpeas.

2. In a food processor, combine the chickpeas, tahini, olive oil, lemon juice, basil, salt, and pepper and pulse until smooth.

3. Serve with the carrots, celery sticks, cucumber slices, and pita chips.

4. Leftover hummus can be stored in the refrigerator in an airtight container for up to 3 days.

PER SERVING (¼ CUP, HUMMUS ONLY): Calories: 188; Total Fat: 8g; Saturated Fat: 1g; Carbohydrates: 22g; Fiber: 7g; Protein: 8g

PEACH AND AVOCADO SALSA

**SERVES 16; PREP TIME: 10 MINUTES
COOK TIME: NONE**

Juicy peaches make the most amazing salsa. Get in some extra doses of fruit and veggies in a whole new way. Serve this salsa over a piece of grilled fish at dinner or with whole-grain tortilla chips for a healthy and satisfying snack.

3 peaches, chopped

½ red bell pepper, chopped

2 scallions, finely chopped

1 avocado, diced

Juice of 1 lime

3 tablespoons chopped fresh cilantro

¼ teaspoon kosher salt

1. In a large bowl, combine the peaches, bell pepper, scallions, avocado, lime juice, cilantro, and salt and toss gently to combine.

2. Serve immediately, or refrigerate in an airtight container for up to 2 days

PER SERVING (¼ CUP): Calories: 32; Total Fat 3g; Saturated Fat: 1g; Carbohydrates: 4g; Fiber: 2g; Protein: 1g

POMEGRANATE GUACAMOLE

**SERVES 4; PREP TIME: 5 MINUTES
COOK TIME: NONE**

Sweet and crunchy pomegranate seeds jazz up this guac in a fabulously simple way. Avocados provide lots of folate, vitamin K, and potassium, very important nutrients during pregnancy.

2 large Hass avocados, peeled, pitted, and diced

¼ cup pomegranate seeds

Fresh lime juice

¼ teaspoon sea salt

In a medium bowl, toss the avocados, pomegranate seeds, and lime juice. Add the salt and stir gently to combine. Serve immediately.

PER SERVING: Calories: 123; Total Fat: 11g; Saturated Fat: 1g; Carbohydrates: 8g; Fiber: 5g; Protein: 2g

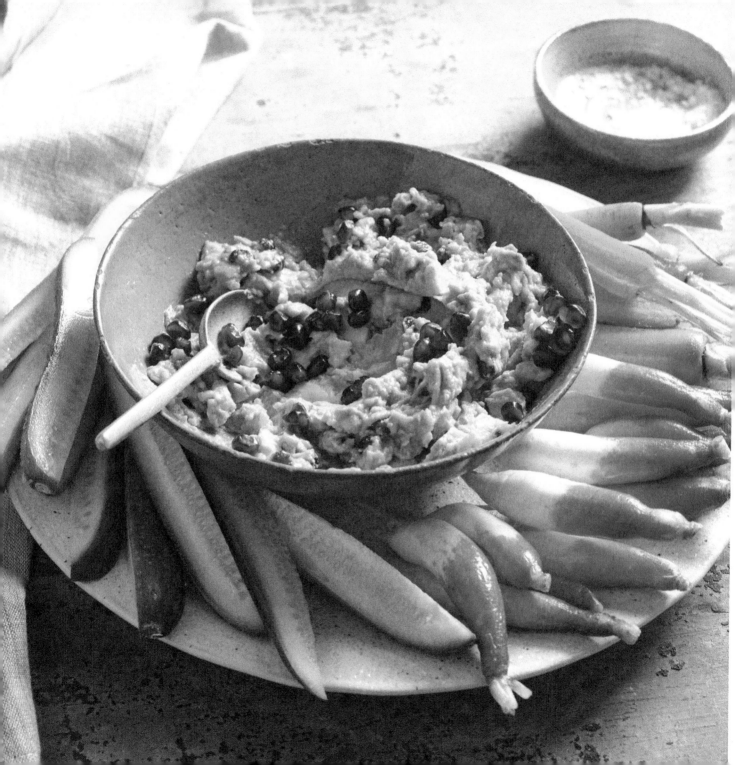

BANANA-COCONUT BITES

SERVES 1; PREP TIME: 5 MINUTES
COOK TIME: NONE

These bite-size treats are better than candy and will help you feel energized and satisfied between meals or for a late night snack. You'll feel like you're eating a decadent treat, but you're getting in a serving of fruit and a dose of healthy fat.

1 medium banana, cut into 5 large slices

2 tablespoons peanut butter

Dried coconut chips

Spread each banana slice with peanut butter and sprinkle with coconut chips.

TIP: If you can't find coconut chips, use dried unsweetened coconut or even some pepitas (shelled pumpkin seeds) for the crunch.

PER SERVING: Calories: 293; Total Fat: 18g; Saturated Fat: 3g; Carbohydrates: 34g; Fiber: 5g; Protein: 10g

HOMEMADE ALMOND BUTTER

SERVES 16; PREP TIME: 5 MINUTES
COOK TIME: NONE

Once you see how easy (and delicious) the home-made version is, you'll probably never buy a jar of almond butter again. Many store-bought nut butters contain additives and stabilizers, but there are none in this recipe. Store in the refrigerator, then bring to room temperature and stir well before each use.

2 cups roasted almonds

Sea salt

Place the almonds in a food processor or high-speed blender. Pulse, then blend until the mixture is the desired consistency. Store in an airtight container.

PER SERVING (1 TABLESPOON): Calories: 69; Total Fat: 6g; Saturated Fat: 0g; Carbohydrates: 2.5g; Fiber: 1.5g; Protein: 3g

AVOCADO-HEMP SPREAD

SERVES 4; PREP TIME: 10 MINUTES
COOK TIME: NONE

Hemp seeds are beyond underappreciated. They add wonderful texture and bite, plus they're filled with protein, fiber, and minerals like magnesium and potassium. They also contain those essential omega-3 fatty acids. Make a batch of this creamy spread and serve with cucumber slices or brown rice crackers for some crunch.

2 large ripe avocados

2 tablespoons hemp seeds

Juice and zest of 1 lime

Pinch of sea salt

1. Cut the avocado in half, discard the seed, and scoop out the flesh into a large bowl.

2. Using a potato masher, mash the avocado until smooth. For an extra-creamy version, use a food processor or high-speed blender.

3. Using a spatula, fold in the hemp seeds, lime juice and zest, and a pinch of sea salt.

4. Serve immediately.

TIP: To make this recipe ahead of time, you can pour a thin layer of water on top and then cover with a tight fitting layer of plastic wrap. The avocado is high in healthy fat and will not absorb the water, but this approach will prevent the mixture from turning brown. When ready to use, remove the plastic, drain the water, and give the mixture a stir.

PER SERVING: Calories: 142; Total Fat: 13g; Saturated Fat: 2g; Carbohydrates: 8g; Fiber: 5g; Protein: 3g

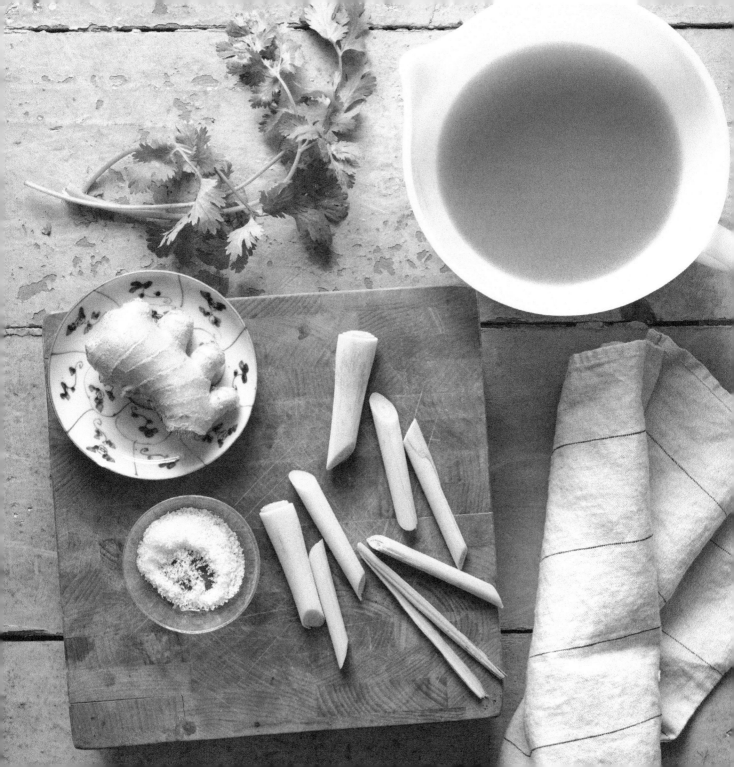

nine

SOUPS AND STEWS

REAL DEAL CHICKEN STOCK

MAKES 3 QUARTS; PREP TIME: 15 MINUTES
COOK TIME: 3 HOURS

Sure, you can buy boxed or canned chicken stock, but nothing tastes as good as the homemade version. Use this same method with the leftover carcass of a roasted or rotisserie chicken you've stored in your freezer up to 3 months.

1 (4-pound) chicken

1 white onion, quartered

2 large carrots, roughly chopped

1 large parsnip, roughly chopped

2 large celery stalks, roughly chopped

2 garlic cloves

1 bunch fresh parsley

10 sprigs fresh thyme

1 tablespoon kosher salt

2 dried bay leaves

1 gallon water, plus more if needed

1. Place the chicken in a large stockpot.

2. Add the onion, carrots, parsnip, celery, garlic, parsley, thyme, salt, and bay leaves.

3. Add enough of the water to cover.

4. Over high heat, bring to a boil uncovered. Reduce the heat to medium-low, and simmer for 3 hours.

5. Strain the stock, discard the chicken and vegetables, and pour into airtight storage containers.

6. Store in the refrigerator for up to 1 week or in the freezer for up to 3 months.

PER SERVING (1 CUP): Calories: 35; Total Fat: 2g; Saturated Fat 1g; Carbohydrates: 0g; Fiber: 0g; Protein: 4g

VEGGIE SCRAP BROTH

MAKES: 1-2 QUARTS; PREP TIME: 5 MINUTES
COOK TIME: 25 MINUTES

Reduce waste and make a delicious base for soups and sauces. Keep a large resealable bag in the freezer for veggie scraps left over from daily cooking. When the bag is full, make a batch of vegetable broth.

Vegetable scraps, like onions, carrots, celery, and herbs

2 garlic cloves

1 bay leaf

1 teaspoon peppercorns

2 teaspoons kosher salt

1. Place the vegetable scraps, garlic, bay leaf, peppercorns, and salt in a large stockpot.

2. Add enough water to cover and bring to a boil over high heat.

3. Lower the heat, and simmer until the liquid is reduced by half.

4. Strain and discard the vegetables, and transfer to airtight containers.

5. Store in the refrigerator for up to 1 week or in the freezer for up to 3 months.

PER SERVING (1 CUP): Calories: 15; Total Fat: 0g; Saturated Fat: 0g; Carbohydrates: 3g; Fiber: 1g; Protein: 0g

GINGER-LEMONGRASS BROTH

MAKES 1 QUART; PREP TIME: 5 MINUTES
COOK TIME: 25 MINUTES

The aroma of this soup will calm your nerves and the ginger infusion will calm your stomach. Use this recipe as a base broth for other soups or sip it plain to help stay hydrated. This is soup for the soul—and the belly.

5 cups vegetable broth (homemade or reduced sodium)

1 (2-inch) piece peeled fresh ginger

2 lemongrass stalks

1 bunch fresh cilantro

1 teaspoon kosher salt

1. In a large soup pot over high heat, combine the broth, ginger, lemongrass, cilantro, and salt.

2. Bring the mixture to a boil. Reduce the heat to low and simmer for 20 minutes.

3. Allow the broth to cool slightly, then strain. Pour into airtight containers.

4. Store in the refrigerator for up to 1 week or in the freezer for up to 3 months.

PER SERVING (1 CUP): Calories: 18; Total Fat: 1g; Saturated Fat: 0g; Carbohydrates: 4g; Fiber: 1g; Protein: 0g

QUICK TOMATO SOUP

SERVES 1; PREP TIME: 5 MINUTES
COOK TIME: 10 MINUTES

A hearty soup doesn't need to take hours to make. Rich in antioxidants like vitamin C and lycopene, this soup tastes better than anything from a can. A splash of cashew milk to finish gives this soup a creamy texture and a decadent taste.

¼ cup marinara sauce (preferably homemade, see page 182)

2 cups low-sodium chicken or vegetable broth

2 tablespoons cashew milk

1. Combine the marinara sauce and broth in a medium saucepan, and bring to a boil over medium-high heat

2. Reduce the heat to medium-low and simmer for 5 minutes

3. Remove from the heat and stir in the cashew milk.

4. Serve warm or at room temperature.

PER SERVING: Calories: 58; Total Fat: 2g; Saturated Fat: 0g; Carbohydrates: 7g; Fiber: 1g; Protein: 3g

COCONUT SOUP

SERVES 4; PREP TIME: 5 MINUTES
COOK TIME: 20 MINUTES

This soup is filled with nutrients and flavor. Combine Ginger-Lemongrass Broth with creamy coconut milk for a Thai-inspired soup that's better for you than any takeout order. And it's so delicious.

1 recipe Ginger-Lemongrass Broth (page 129)

1 (14-ounce) can unsweetened full-fat coconut milk

2 tablespoons hoisin sauce

1 cup sliced mushrooms

2 tablespoons chopped scallions

Rice noodles, cooked (about 2 cups)

Chopped fresh cilantro, for serving

1. In a large soup pot, bring the broth to a simmer over medium-high heat.

2. Add the coconut milk, hoisin sauce, mushrooms, scallions, and noodles and stir to combine.

3. Return to a simmer, reduce the heat to medium, and continue to simmer for 10 to 12 minutes.

4. Serve garnished with fresh cilantro.

TIP: Try using brown rice noodles for some extra whole grains.

PER SERVING: Calories: 356; Total Fat: 24g; Saturated Fat: 21g; Carbohydrates: 32g; Fiber: 4g; Protein: 4g

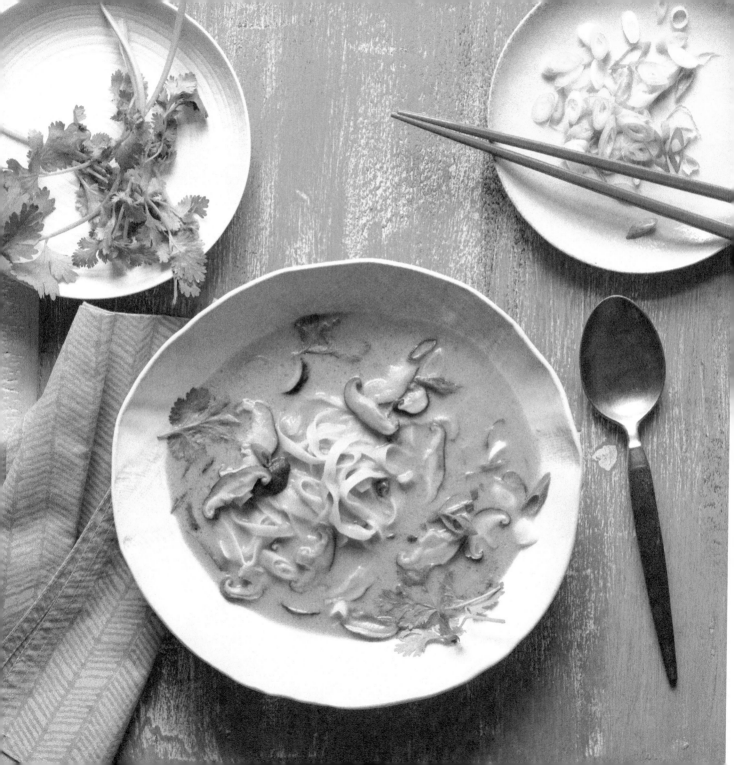

QUICK AND EASY MINESTRONE

**SERVES 4; PREP TIME: 10 MINUTES
COOK TIME: 30 MINUTES**

Beans, veggies, and pasta make minestrone a warm and satisfying one-pot meal. This combination of ingredients has folate, iron, protein, fluids, and electrolytes—everything a healthy mom-to-be needs.

1 tablespoon olive oil

½ cup finely chopped onion

1 large carrot, chopped

3 cups low-sodium vegetable or chicken broth

1 can diced tomatoes

1 (15-ounce) can kidney beans, drained and rinsed

Kosher salt

Freshly ground black pepper

½ cup whole-wheat pasta

2 cups baby spinach

Parmesan cheese, grated, for serving (optional)

1. Heat the olive oil in a medium soup pot over medium-high heat.

2. Add the onion and carrot and sauté until tender, about 5 minutes.

3. Add the broth, diced tomatoes, and beans. Season with salt and pepper, and stir to combine. Bring to a simmer.

4. Add the pasta, stirring frequently. When the soup comes to a simmer, reduce the heat to medium-low and cook for 15 minutes or until the pasta is just tender.

5. Just before serving, stir in the spinach and top with Parmesan cheese (if desired).

TIP: For a gluten-free alternative, try a quinoa pasta in this recipe.

PER SERVING: Calories: 338; Total Fat: 6g; Saturated Fat: 1g; Carbohydrates: 53g; Fiber: 12g; Protein: 20g

SPEEDY BROCCOLI AND CHEDDAR SOUP

SERVES 4; PREP TIME: 15 MINUTES
COOK TIME: 15 MINUTES

This creamy soup is perfect for a weeknight dinner with a salad and some whole-grain crackers. It also freezes well, so make extra to have on hand for when the baby arrives.

2 tablespoons olive oil

½ white onion, chopped

Kosher salt

Freshly ground black pepper

4 cups chopped broccoli (florets and stems)

2 cups homemade or low-sodium chicken or vegetable broth

1 cup whole milk

1 cup shredded Cheddar cheese

1. In a medium saucepan, heat the oil over medium-high heat, add the onion, season with salt and pepper, and sauté for 2 to 3 minutes.

2. Add the broccoli, broth, and milk, and heat until simmering. Remove from the heat.

3. Add the cheese and purée the soup to the desired consistency using an immersion blender (or a countertop blender or food processor).

4. Serve hot.

TIP: Having boxed chicken broth or vegetable broth on hand is a huge time-saver. Get the low-sodium varieties and add more kosher salt if needed.

PER SERVING: Calories: 254; Total Fat: 19g; Saturated Fat: 8g; Carbohydrates: 11g; Fiber: 3g; Protein: 12g

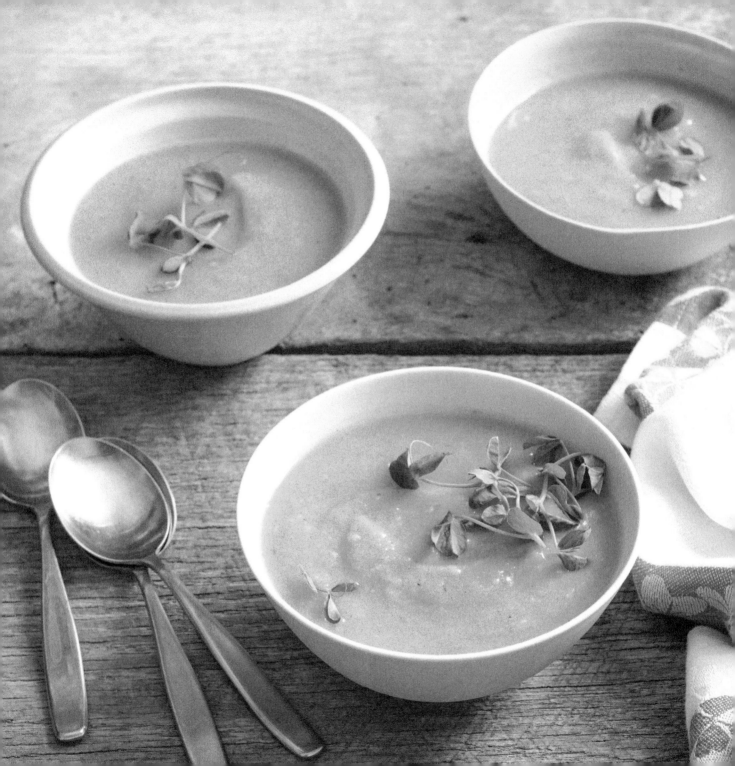

ROASTED VEGETABLE SOUP

SERVES 8; PREP TIME: 15 MINUTES
COOK TIME: 50 MINUTES

Make roasted veggies as a dinner side dish and turn leftovers into this creamy and delicious soup. Chop the vegetables into equal-size chunks for even cooking. This soup also freezes beautifully.

1 small butternut squash (about 2 pounds), peeled, seeded, and diced

1 medium onion, chopped

1 red bell pepper, chopped

10 ounces potatoes, peeled and chopped

2 medium parsnips, peeled and chopped

2 tablespoons olive oil

1 teaspoon kosher salt

Freshly ground black pepper

6 Veggie Scrap Broth (page 129)

1. Preheat the oven to 400°F.

2. Spread the squash, onion, bell pepper, potatoes, and parsnips in a large baking pan.

3. Drizzle with olive oil, season with salt and pepper, and toss to combine.

4. Roast for 30 to 40 minutes or until fork-tender.

5. Transfer to a large soup pot and add the vegetable broth.

6. Purée the mixture with an immersion blender (or use a countertop blender or food processor). Reheat over medium heat until hot, stirring frequently. Serve.

PER SERVING (1 CUP): Calories: 141; Total Fat 4g; Saturated Fat: 1g; Carbohydrates: 27g; Fiber: 5g; Protein: 2g

COD AND FENNEL STEW

SERVES 2; PREP TIME: 10 MINUTES
COOK TIME: 40 MINUTES

Fennel, tomatoes, and a light white fish like cod are a brilliant flavor combination, and fennel works as a natural digestive aid. Reserve some of the feathery green fennel fronds to garnish the stew. To take this stew to another level, stir in a pinch of saffron.

2 tablespoons extra-virgin olive oil

1 medium red onion, chopped

1 medium green bell pepper, chopped

1 bulb fennel, finely chopped

3 garlic cloves, minced

½ teaspoon kosher salt

2 (14-ounce) cans diced tomatoes

3 cups low-sodium vegetable broth

¾ pound cod, cut into bite-size chunks

3 cups chopped fresh Swiss chard

1. Heat the olive oil in a large soup pot over medium-high heat.

2. Add the onion, bell pepper, and fennel, reduce the heat to medium, and sauté until softened, about 10 minutes.

3. Add the garlic, salt, tomatoes, and broth. Bring the mixture to a simmer and cook for about 15 minutes.

4. Add the cod and Swiss chard and cook until the fish is opaque, about 5 minutes.

5. Serve immediately. Store leftovers in an airtight container in the refrigerator for up to 2 days.

TIP: Cod is a high-protein, lowfat fish. Ask your fishmonger for wild cod and refer to sustainability guides such as Seafood Watch to determine the best seafood choices.

PER SERVING: Calories: 472; Total Fat: 17g; Saturated Fat: 2g; Carbohydrates: 27g; Fiber: 8g; Protein: 51g

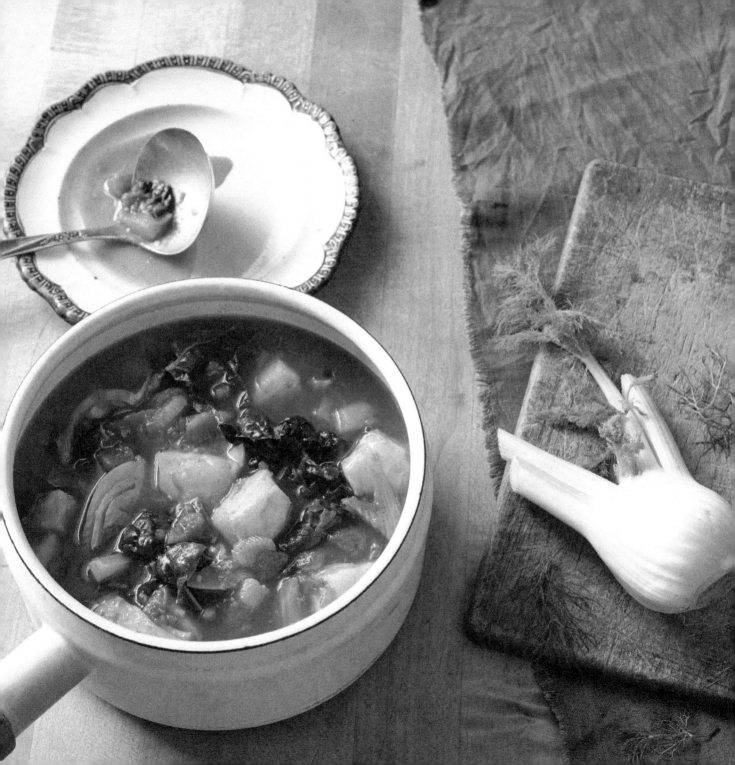

SLOW COOKER LENTIL SOUP

SERVES 6; PREP TIME: 5 MINUTES
COOK TIME: 8 HOURS OR OVERNIGHT

Lentils are a superfood, rich in fiber for digestion, iron to combat anemia, and other minerals. Toss the ingredients in the slow cooker in the morning and the soup will be ready by dinnertime.

2 cups dried lentils

3 tablespoons olive oil

2 garlic cloves, chopped

2 cups chopped carrots

2 tablespoons tomato paste

2 teaspoons kosher salt

½ tablespoon freshly ground black pepper

2 teaspoons herbes de Provence

6 cups low-sodium chicken stock or vegetable broth

1. Combine all the ingredients in a slow cooker.

2. Cover and set on high for 8 hours.

3. Serve with a side salad lightly dressed with balsamic vinaigrette.

TIP: To make the side salad, combine some dark leafy lettuce with fresh veggies like shredded carrots and sliced bell peppers. Dress it with a light drizzle of Basic Vinaigrette Dressing (page 156) using balsamic vinegar.

PER SERVING: Calories: 318; Total Fat: 8g; Saturated Fat: 2g; Carbohydrates: 53g; Fiber: 14g; Protein: 16g

SLOW COOKER CHICKEN STEW

SERVES 4; PREP TIME: 5 MINUTES
COOK TIME: 8 HOURS OR OVERNIGHT

This dish is a set-it-and-forget-it wonder meal for busy days. Leftovers are also great for lunch the next day. If you really want to plan ahead, combine the ingredients (except for the spinach) in a resealable bag and store in the freezer. Just toss the frozen ingredients in the slow cooker and cook, stirring in the fresh spinach before serving. Serve with whole-grain pasta or brown rice.

1 pound boneless, skinless chicken thighs

Kosher salt

Freshly ground black pepper

1 (14-ounce) can diced tomatoes

1 (15-ounce) can reduced-sodium white beans, drained and rinsed

1 teaspoon dried thyme

6 cups fresh baby spinach

1. Season the chicken pieces on both sides with salt and pepper.

2. Put the chicken, tomatoes, beans, and thyme in the slow cooker. Cover and cook on low for 8 hours.

3. Before serving, shred the chicken and mix in the spinach.

PER SERVING: Calories: 281; Total Fat 5g; Saturated Fat: 1g; Carbohydrates: 28g; Fiber: 7g; Protein: 32g

SIX-INGREDIENT CHILI

SERVES 4; PREP TIME: 10 MINUTES
COOK TIME: 30 MINUTES

Chili is a dish that's filled with nutritious ingredients and lots of flavor. An amazing chili doesn't have to be complicated and this recipe proves it. Make it as mild or as spicy as you want. Freeze leftovers in a resealable bag for a tasty meal after baby arrives.

½ pound ground turkey

½ large white onion, finely chopped

1 poblano or jalapeño chile pepper, roughly chopped

¼ teaspoon kosher salt

2 teaspoons chili powder (adjust as needed)

1 (14-ounce) can diced tomatoes

1 (15-ounce) can red kidney beans, drained and rinsed

1. Place the ground turkey, onion, and chile pepper in a large pot over medium heat, and sauté until the turkey is browned and vegetables are tender, about 10 minutes.

2. Season with salt and chili powder, and stir well.

3. Stir in the diced tomatoes and beans, and bring to a rapid simmer.

4. Reduce the heat to low and simmer uncovered, stirring occasionally, for 20 minutes.

5. Serve with desired toppings (see Tip).

TIP: To make this chili vegetarian, replace the ground turkey with an additional can of beans and some diced sweet potatoes. Increase cooking time about 20 minutes or until the sweet potatoes are fork-tender.

TIP: Toppings for chili can include fresh cilantro, lime wedges, a dollop of Greek yogurt, some crushed corn tortilla chips, and sliced black olives.

PER SERVING (WITHOUT TOPPINGS): Calories: 200; Total Fat: 5g; Saturated Fat: 1g; Carbohydrates: 23g; Fiber: 7g; Protein: 16g

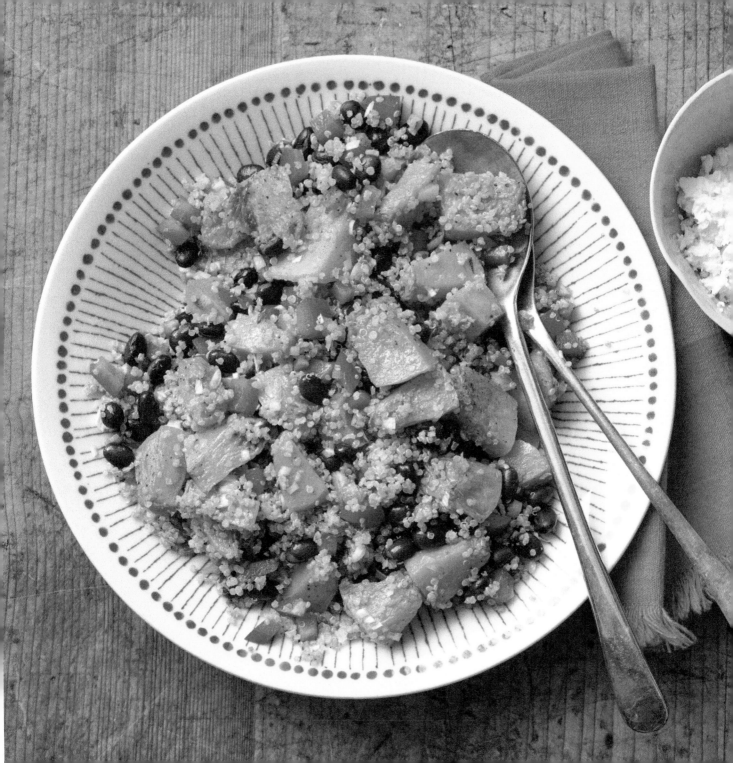

TWO-BEAN SALAD

SERVES 4; PREP TIME: 10 MINUTES, PLUS 1 HOUR
SITTING TIME; COOK TIME: NONE

There's just something about the combo of these simple flavors and textures that's mind blowing: creamy beans, sweet peppers, crunchy celery, topped off with a tangy dressing. Add some cooked brown rice or quinoa for an even more satisfying meal.

1 (15-ounce) can kidney beans, drained and rinsed

1 (15-ounce) can cannellini beans, drained and rinsed

1 cup finely chopped celery

1 cup finely chopped green bell pepper

2 tablespoons chopped fresh parsley

Basic Vinaigrette Dressing (page 156)

1. In a large bowl, add the kidney beans, cannellini beans, celery, bell pepper, parsley, and vinaigrette. Toss well.

2. Allow the mixture to sit for at least 1 hour for flavors to develop.

3. Serve chilled or at room temperature.

PER SERVING: Calories: 258; Total Fat: 6g; Saturated Fat: 1g; Carbohydrates: 39g; Fiber: 11g; Protein: 13g

How to Cook Dried Beans

Canned beans are convenient and affordable, but dried beans are the most budget-friendly. With a little planning, dried beans are also incredibly easy to prepare. Soak the beans in a bowl of water overnight in the refrigerator. When ready to cook, rinse, drain, and put in a large stock pot with enough water to cover by 2 to 3 inches. Bring to a boil over medium-high heat. Reduce the heat to low, and simmer until the beans are fork-tender, approximately 40 to 50 minutes, depending on the type of bean.

You can infuse the cooking liquid with extra flavor by adding a bay leaf or other fresh herbs. You can season with salt, but wait until the beans are almost done cooking. Adding salt too early in the cooking process can make the beans tough.

WILD RICE SALAD

**SERVES 2; PREP TIME: 10 MINUTES, PLUS 1 HOUR
SITTING TIME; COOK TIME: 35 MINUTES**

*This four-ingredient recipe is ready in minutes.
It's elegant enough for a dinner party, and also
makes a delightful accompaniment to a week-
night dinner. Wild rice offers a wide array of
nutrients not found in whole-grain brown rice,
including more folate and vitamin B6.*

1 cup wild rice

Kosher salt

1 Granny Smith apple, finely chopped

¼ cup chopped walnuts

Basic Vinaigrette Dressing (page 156)

1. Combine the rice with 2 cups of water and
   a pinch of salt in a medium saucepan over
   medium-high heat. Bring to a boil, reduce
   the heat to low, and simmer, covered, until
   the water is absorbed and the rice is tender,
   about 30 minutes.

2. Put the rice, apple, and walnuts in a large
   salad bowl. Add the vinaigrette and toss well
   to combine.

3. Allow the mixture to sit for at least 1 hour for
   flavors to develop.

PER SERVING: Calories: 420; Total Fat: 16g; Saturated
Fat: 2g; Carbohydrates: 74g; Fiber: 8g; Protein: 16g

ARUGULA SALAD

SERVES 1; PREP TIME: 10 MINUTES
COOK TIME: NONE

Peppery arugula, walnuts, and sweet-tart cranberries come together to create a delicious leafy green salad that offers vital nutrients for pregnancy, including iron, omega-3 fats, vitamins, and inflammation-fighting antioxidants.

1 tablespoon extra-virgin olive oil

2 teaspoons balsamic vinegar

1 teaspoon honey

¼ teaspoon Dijon mustard

Kosher salt

Freshly ground black pepper

3 cups arugula

2 tablespoons chopped walnuts

2 tablespoons crumbled feta cheese

1 tablespoon dried cranberries

1. In a large bowl, combine the olive oil, balsamic vinegar, honey, and mustard.

2. Season with salt and pepper. Whisk together well.

3. Add the arugula, walnuts, feta, and cranberries. Toss well to combine. Serve.

PER SERVING: Calories: 309; Total Fat: 27g; Saturated Fat: 6g; Carbohydrates: 11g; Fiber: 2g; Protein: 8g

SESAME CHICKEN SALAD

SERVES 1; PREP TIME: 10 MINUTES
COOK TIME: NONE

Sweet, savory, tangy, crunchy—this salad will satisfy just about any craving. Add whatever protein you have in the fridge. If you want to make this vegetarian, grilled vegetables, tofu, or shelled edamame can be your protein.

3 cups mixed greens

4 ounces cooked chicken breast, shredded

2 tablespoons slivered almonds

½ cup sliced cucumber

1 cup fresh orange segments

2 scallions, chopped

Sesame Ginger Dressing (page 156)

1. Combine all the ingredients in a large bowl and toss well.

2. Serve immediately, or refrigerate in an airtight container for up to 2 days.

PER SERVING: Calories: 416; Total Fat 20g; Saturated Fat: 3g; Carbohydrates: 16g; Fiber: 4g; Protein: 40g

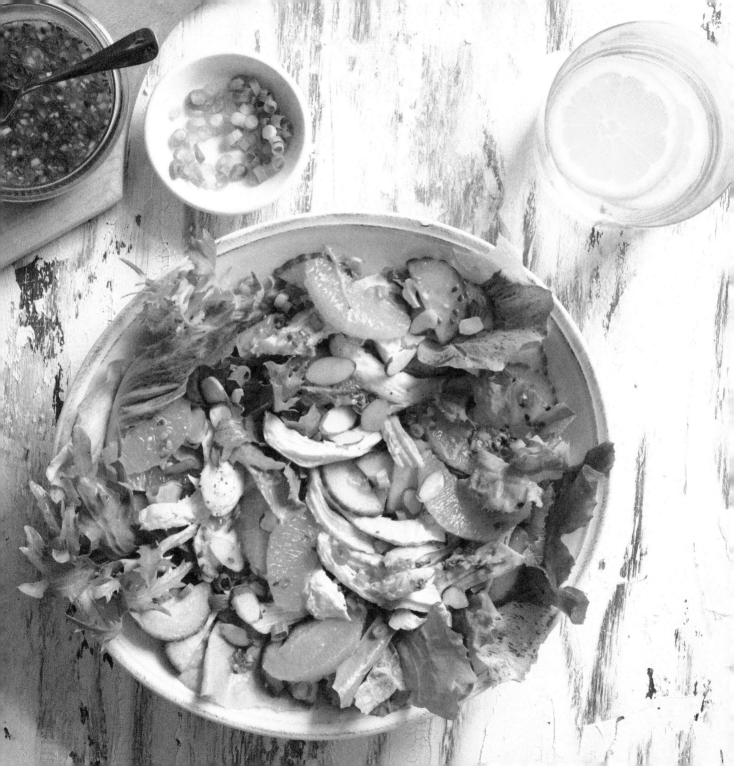

BUTTERNUT SQUASH AND QUINOA SALAD

SERVES 6; PREP TIME: 15 MINUTES
COOK TIME: 30 MINUTES

Roasted butternut squash is a sinfully sweet root veggie but guilt-free. Make a large batch of this oven-roasted squash as a dinner side dish and then save some of the leftovers for making this salad.

2 cups peeled diced butternut squash

3 tablespoons extra-virgin olive oil, divided

Kosher salt

Freshly ground black pepper

1 cup quinoa

1 (15-ounce) can black beans, drained and rinsed

1 cup diced red bell pepper

3 scallions, finely chopped

Freshly squeezed lime juice to taste

½ cup crumbled lowfat feta cheese (optional)

1. Preheat the oven to 400°F.

2. Toss the squash with 1 tablespoon of the olive oil, and season with salt and pepper.

3. Roast until fork-tender, about 30 minutes.

4. In a medium saucepan over medium-high heat, combine the quinoa with 2 cups of water and cook, covered, for 15 minutes until the water is absorbed and the quinoa is tender.

5. In a large salad bowl, put the squash, quinoa, black beans, bell pepper, scallions, remaining 2 tablespoons of the olive oil, lime juice, and feta cheese (if using) and toss to combine. Serve.

PER SERVING: Calories: 287; Total Fat: 10g; Saturated Fat: 1g; Carbohydrates: 32g; Fiber: 5g; Protein: 7g

COBB PASTA SALAD

SERVES 4; PREP TIME: 10 MINUTES
COOK TIME: NONE

This salad is a new spin on a classic salad. It is a great way to satisfy a craving for pasta without going overboard on calories. Experiment with different types of pasta, and for a lowfat take on the bacon found in the traditional Cobb salad recipe, add some marinated tempeh to the mix.

   4 cups cooked whole-grain pasta

   2 hard-boiled eggs, chopped

   1 cup sliced cucumber

   1 cup chopped tomato

   1 cup diced avocado

   ½ cup lowfat salad dressing

   12 cups chopped romaine lettuce

1. Combine all the ingredients in a large bowl and toss well.

2. Serve immediately.

PER SERVING: Calories: 267; Total Fat: 7g; Saturated Fat: 1g; Carbohydrates: 42g; Fiber: 7g; Protein: 9g

KALE AND MANGO SALAD

SERVES 2; PREP TIME: 10 MINUTES
COOK TIME: NONE

Lacinato kale, also known as dinosaur kale, is a variety with flat, dark green leaves. It's full of antioxidants and more tender. The bitter green is a nice contrast to the tangy fresh mango and this salad is filled with vitamins A, C, and K for healthy skin and blood.

   2 tablespoons extra-virgin olive oil

   2 teaspoons red wine vinegar

   2 teaspoons honey

   2 teaspoons minced shallot

   Kosher salt

   Freshly ground black pepper

   6 cups chopped lacinato kale

   1 cup diced mango

1. In a large bowl, combine the olive oil, vinegar, honey, and shallot.

2. Season with salt and pepper, and whisk the dressing well.

3. Add the kale and mango, toss, and serve.

PER SERVING: Calories: 292; Total Fat: 16g; Saturated Fat: 2g; Carbohydrates: 36g; Fiber: 9g; Protein: 6g

FIESTA CHICKEN SALAD

SERVES 1; PREP TIME: 10 MINUTES
COOK TIME: NONE

A simple lime juice and olive oil dressing plus a kick from salsa elevate this salad from ordinary to fabulous. This recipe is also delicious using baby spinach or arugula instead of lettuce, or wrapped in a warm corn tortilla.

3 cups mixed salad greens

1 medium grilled chicken breast, sliced

½ avocado, diced

2 tablespoons salsa

2 tablespoons shredded cheese (optional)

½ cup chopped tomato

2 teaspoons olive oil

Fresh lime juice

1. Put all the ingredients in a large salad bowl, including the cheese (if using), and toss well to combine.

2. Serve immediately.

PER SERVING: Calories: 519; Total Fat: 34g; Saturated Fat: 7g; Carbohydrates: 19g; Fiber: 9g; Protein: 40g

AVOCADO AND BLACK BEAN SALAD

SERVES 4; PREP TIME: 10 MINUTES
COOK TIME: NONE

Like guacamole with the volume turned up, this protein-packed salad gets its punch from tender black beans and a few dashes of hot sauce. The creamy avocado balances out the heat, making the salad flavorful, not spicy.

3 avocados, diced

1 (15-ounce) can black beans, drained and rinsed

1 pint cherry tomatoes, halved

½ teaspoon hot sauce

Juice of 2 limes

¼ teaspoon kosher salt

Mixed salad greens

1. In a medium bowl, combine avocados, beans, and tomatoes.

2. Add hot sauce, lime juice, and salt, and toss gently to mix.

3. Serve the mixture over the salad greens.

PER SERVING: Calories: 273; Total Fat: 16g; Saturated Fat: 2g; Carbohydrates: 28g; Fiber: 15g; Protein: 9g

WALDORF CHICKEN SALAD

SERVES 4; PREP TIME: 10 MINUTES
COOK TIME: NONE

Make this chicken salad for a brunch or lunch for a crowd, maybe even a baby shower? Make a big batch over the weekend, and brown-bag it for lunch during the workweek. Crunchy apples and walnuts add fiber and texture and keep you feeling satisfied all day long.

¼ cup plain yogurt

1 tablespoon apple cider vinegar

¼ teaspoon kosher salt

3 cups skinless roasted chicken, shredded

½ cup chopped celery

1 medium apple, chopped

½ cup chopped walnuts

Mixed salad greens

1. In a large bowl, whisk together the yogurt, vinegar, and salt.

2. Add the chicken, celery, apple, and walnuts, and toss well to coat.

3. Serve on four salad plates over the salad greens.

TIP: For a vegan version of this recipe, replace the chicken with roasted tofu and replace the yogurt with Veganaise, a mayonnaise alternative.

PER SERVING: Calories: 320; Total Fat: 13g; Saturated Fat: 2g; Carbohydrates: 14g; Fiber: 2g; Protein: 36g

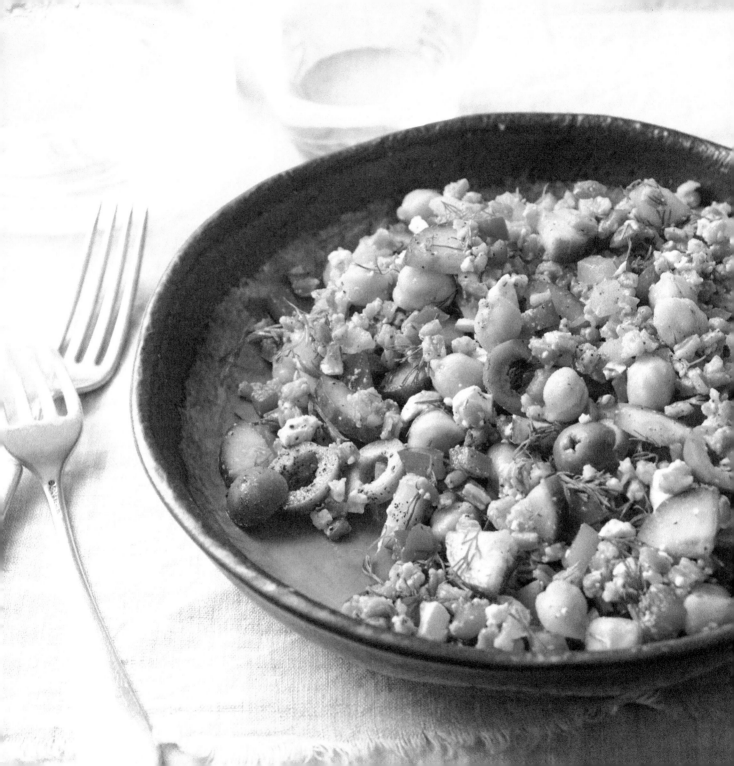

FARRO SALAD

SERVES 4; PREP TIME: 10 MINUTES
COOK TIME: 30 MINUTES

Farro is a whole grain filled with energy-producing B vitamins, fiber, and a distinctive nutty flavor. Add the dressing while the farro is still warm so it can absorb the flavor.

2 teaspoons kosher salt, divided

¾ cup farro

1 tablespoon extra-virgin olive oil

½ teaspoon freshly ground black pepper

½ cup canned chickpeas, drained and rinsed

½ cup diced cucumber

¼ cup diced red bell pepper

¼ cup diced yellow bell pepper

¼ cup sliced olives

¼ cup crumbled feta cheese

2 tablespoons chopped fresh dill

Basic Vinaigrette Dressing (page 156)

1. Bring a large pot of water to a boil and add 1 teaspoon salt.

2. Add the farro and cook according to package directions.

3. Drain, transfer to a large bowl, add the olive oil, the remaining 1 teaspoon salt, and the pepper. Toss well.

4. When cool, add the chickpeas, cucumber, red bell pepper, yellow bell pepper, olives, feta cheese, dill, and vinaigrette. Toss well to combine.

5. Serve at room temperature or chilled.

TIP: Farro does contain gluten, so for an alternative, you can make this salad with quinoa or brown rice.

PER SERVING: Calories: 251; Total Fat: 12g; Saturated Fat: 2g; Carbohydrates: 31g; Fiber: 4g; Protein: 7g

BASIL CHICKEN SALAD

SERVES 6; PREP TIME: 20 MINUTES
COOK TIME: 35 MINUTES

Make this salad for brunch, lunch, or dinner on a hot summer night. You'll love it so much you'll be keeping batches on hand at all times. It also makes a nice gift for a friend who has just had a baby and doesn't have time to cook.

4 large split chicken breasts, bone-in, skin on

Olive oil

Kosher salt

Freshly ground black pepper

2 tablespoons mayonnaise

2 tablespoons plain nonfat Greek yogurt

¾ cup chopped celery

½ cup chopped basil

1. Preheat the oven to 375°F.

2. Place the chicken breasts skin-side up on a baking pan.

3. Drizzle with 3 teaspoons olive oil and season well with salt and pepper.

4. Bake for 35 to 40 minutes or until the internal temperature of the chicken reaches 165°F.

5. When the chicken is cool enough to handle, discard the skin, remove the breast meat from the bones, and chop into bite-size pieces.

6. Transfer the chicken to a large bowl and add the mayonnaise, yogurt, celery, and basil. Season with more salt and pepper, if needed. Toss the salad to mix well.

7. Serve immediately or put in the refrigerator to chill slightly before serving.

PER SERVING: Calories: 225; Total Fat 7g; Saturated Fat: 1.5g; Carbohydrates: 1g; Fiber: 0g; Protein: 36g

CURRIED SQUASH

SERVES 4; PREP TIME: 5 MINUTES
COOK TIME: 25 MINUTES

Many pregnant women crave the smell and flavor of curry. Besides being delicious, curry spices are also rich in nutrients and antioxidants that fight inflammation and help keep cells healthy. Acorn squash is a mild squash with a tender, pleasing texture; if you prefer a sweeter squash, try butternut or Hubbard varieties.

2 medium acorn squash

1 tablespoon olive oil

¼ teaspoon kosher salt

1 teaspoon curry powder

¼ cup chopped cashews

1. Preheat the oven to 425°F.

2. Cut the squash in half, scoop out the seeds, and cut into quarters.

3. Place skin-side down on a baking pan.

4. Drizzle with the olive oil and sprinkle with the salt and curry powder.

5. Roast for 20 to 25 minutes or until fork-tender.

6. Top with the chopped cashews and serve.

TIP: If the thought of curry makes you queasy during your pregnancy, try using Italian seasoning instead (oregano, basil, thyme).

PER SERVING: Calories: 157; Total Fat: 7g; Saturated Fat: 1g; Carbohydrates: 25g; Fiber: 4g; Protein: 3g

CRISPY OVEN FRIES

SERVES 4; PREP TIME: 15 MINUTES
COOK TIME: 35 MINUTES

Pass on greasy takeout and make fries that taste better and are better for you. Potatoes are an important source of potassium, vital for proper heart and muscle function. And don't remove those potato skins; they are overflowing with additional vitamins and minerals.

4 Russet potatoes, scrubbed clean

2 tablespoons olive oil

1 teaspoon fresh thyme

½ teaspoon kosher salt

1. Preheat the oven to 400°F.

2. Cut the potatoes into equal-size fries.

3. Place on a baking pan and toss with the olive oil, thyme, and salt.

4. Bake for 35 to 40 minutes, turning once or twice during the last 15 minutes of cooking.

5. Serve hot.

TIP: Use this method with other root vegetables like sweet potatoes, parsnips, and carrots.

PER SERVING: Calories: 228; Total Fat: 7g; Saturated Fat: 1g; Carbohydrates: 38g; Fiber: 3g; Protein: 5g

CAULIFLOWER RICE

SERVES 4; PREP TIME: 5 MINUTES
COOK TIME: 10 MINUTES

Cauliflower takes on a new life when cut into "rice." Use this basic process to prepare it and add any flavors you like. Suggestions include tamari and ginger, sun-dried tomato and basil, or parsley and lemon zest.

1 head cauliflower, chopped into large pieces

1 tablespoon olive oil

½ teaspoon kosher salt

Freshly ground black pepper

1. Place the cauliflower in a food processor (or blender) and pulse until finely chopped with a texture like rice.

2. Heat the olive oil in a large skillet.

3. Add cauliflower, salt, and season with pepper, and sauté until just tender, about 10 minutes.

PER SERVING: Calories: 82; Total Fat: 4g; Saturated Fat: 1g; Carbohydrates: 10g; Fiber: 4g; Protein: 4g

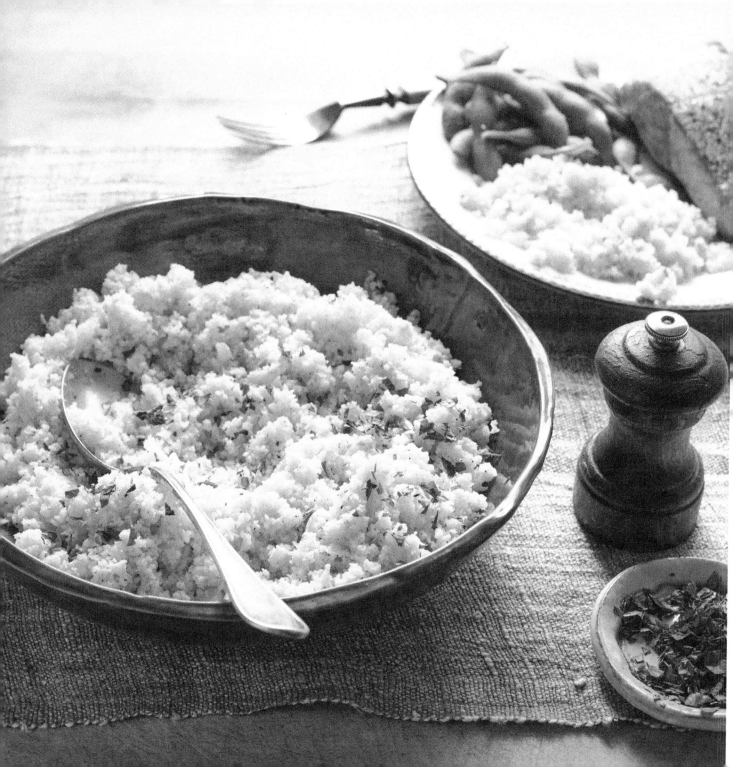

SESAME GINGER DRESSING

MAKES 1 CUP: PREP TIME: 5 MINUTES
COOK TIME: NONE

Homemade dressings are the key to a truly healthy, all-natural salad. Make a new batch each week and store it in the fridge to enjoy with salads or as a marinade for meat, fish, tofu, or tempeh. Since there are no additives, the oil will solidify, so just let it sit on the counter for about 15 minutes before using.

1 tablespoon toasted sesame seeds

1 teaspoon grated peeled fresh ginger

2 tablespoons tamari sauce

2 tablespoons rice vinegar

1 tablespoon honey

1 scallion, finely chopped

Juice of ½ lime

⅓ cup extra-virgin olive oil

¼ cup freshly squeezed orange juice

2 teaspoons toasted sesame oil

1. Combine all the ingredients in a lidded glass jar or other container.

2. Cover and shake well.

3. Store in the refrigerator for up to 1 week.

PER TABLESPOON: Calories: 57; Total Fat: 6g; Saturated Fat: 0g; Carbohydrates: 2g; Fiber: 0g; Protein: 0g

BASIC VINAIGRETTE DRESSING

MAKES ¾ CUP; PREP TIME: 5 MINUTES
COOK TIME: NONE

Follow this recipe for the traditional French salad dressing. For extra flavor, add a pinch of classic herbs: tarragon, thyme, and chives. Make it extra fancy with champagne vinegar or naturally sweet balsamic vinegar

¼ cup red or white wine vinegar

½ cup extra-virgin olive oil

Juice of ½ lemon

1 garlic clove, grated

¼ teaspoon kosher salt

⅛ teaspoon freshly ground black pepper

1. Combine all the ingredients in a sealable glass jar or container.

2. Cover and shake well.

3. Store in the refrigerator for up to 1 week.

PER TABLESPOON: Calories: 80; Total Fat: 9g; Saturated Fat: 1g; Carbohydrates: 1g; Fiber: 0g; Protein: 0g

FRESH RASPBERRY DRESSING

MAKES 1 CUP; PREP TIME: 5 MINUTES
COOK TIME: NONE

Fresh raspberries make for a salad dressing richly laced with vitamin C and antioxidants. Try with strawberries or blackberries, too.

½ cup fresh raspberries

2 tablespoons freshly squeezed lemon juice

½ cup extra-virgin olive oil

2 tablespoons red wine vinegar

1 tablespoon chopped scallion

Pinch kosher salt

Freshly ground black pepper

1. Place all the ingredients in a blender and blend until smooth.

2. Store in the refrigerator for up to 1 week.

PER TABLESPOON: Calories: 65; Total Fat: 7g; Saturated Fat: 0g; Carbohydrates: 1g; Fiber: 0g; Protein: 0g

CREAMY MISO YOGURT DRESSING

MAKES ⅔ CUP; PREP TIME: 5 MINUTES
COOK TIME: NONE

Never underestimate the power of fermented soybean paste. Miso not only adds savory flavor, but it also helps promote a healthy digestive system with its probiotic content. To make this recipe dairy-free, use a cultured nondairy milk product or ¼ cup of soy milk.

½ cup lowfat plain kefir or Greek yogurt

Juice of ½ lemon

3 tablespoons extra-virgin olive oil

1 garlic clove, minced

2 tablespoons miso paste

¼ teaspoon kosher salt

1. Place all the ingredients in a blender and blend until smooth.

2. Use immediately or store in the refrigerator for up to 1 week.

PER TABLESPOON: Calories: 44; Total Fat: 4g; Saturated Fat: 0g; Carbohydrates: 1g; Fiber: 0g; Protein: 1g

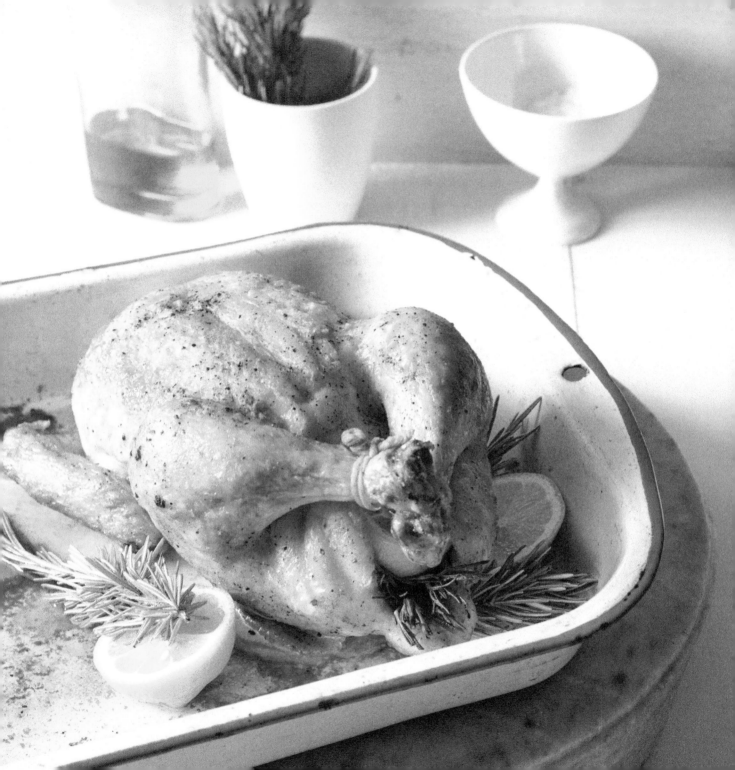

SALMON SALAD COLLARD WRAPS

**SERVES 2; PREP TIME: 15 MINUTES
COOK TIME: 30 SECONDS**

Once you try a collards wrap, you'll never feel the same way about sandwiches again. This wrap is a wonderfully healthy gluten-free option. You can also make this omega-3 rich salmon salad with any kind of tortilla or bread, or serve it over a bed of mixed greens.

1 large collard leaf, stem removed

3 ounces cooked salmon

1 tablespoons Greek yogurt

1 teaspoon Dijon mustard

2 tablespoons chopped fresh celery

2 teaspoons chopped fresh dill

1. Blanch the collard leaf in a large pot of boiling water for 30 seconds.

2. Remove and transfer to a bowl of ice water to set the color. Remove from the water, pat dry, and set aside on a plate.

3. In a medium bowl, combine the salmon, yogurt, mustard, celery, and dill.

4. Mix the salad together gently and place in the middle of the collard leaf.

5. To wrap the leaf around the salad burrito style: fold the left side over the salmon, then the right side. To finish, roll the leaf up from the bottom.

6. Cut in half and serve.

TIP: Blanched collard leaves can be prepared up to 2 days in advance and stored in the refrigerator. Lay them flat between damp paper towels.

PER SERVING: Calories: 176; Total Fat: 7g; Saturated Fat: 1g; Carbohydrates: 3g; Fiber: 2g; Protein: 24g

ALMOND SALMON CAKES

SERVES 2; PREP TIME: 15 MINUTES
COOK TIME: 20 MINUTES

Canned salmon is an underappreciated protein source. It's affordable, easy to find, and super easy to prepare.

2 (5-ounce) cans salmon, drained

1 egg, beaten

Pinch red pepper flakes

¼ cup almond flour

2 tablespoons olive oil, divided

Lemon wedges, for serving

1. Preheat the oven to 375°F.

2. In a medium bowl, combine the salmon, egg, red pepper flakes, almond flour, and 1 tablespoon of the olive oil. Mix together with a fork.

3. Form the mixture into 4 patties.

4. Transfer to a baking sheet and brush with the remaining 1 tablespoon olive oil.

5. Bake for 20 minutes, turning once halfway through the cooking, until golden brown.

6. Serve with lemon wedges.

TIP: You can also make this recipe with pulverized rice cracker crumbs instead of almond flour.

PER SERVING: Calories: 416; Total Fat: 31g; Saturated Fat: 5g; Carbohydrates: 3g; Fiber: 1g; Protein: 35g

TOFU STIR-FRY

SERVES 4; PREP TIME: 15 MINUTES
COOK TIME: 10 MINUTES

Feeling too tired to cook? This quick and healthy stir-fry featuring protein-packed tofu and fresh veggies cooks up in minutes and will keep your stomach feeling satisfied and content for hours.

1 tablespoon coconut oil

1 garlic clove, minced

1-inch piece peeled fresh ginger, minced

1 pound extra-firm tofu, drained and cut into cubes

4 cups broccoli florets

1 medium red bell pepper, cut into strips

1 cup thinly sliced carrot rounds

½ red onion, sliced

2 tablespoons gluten-free tamari sauce

Cooked brown rice, for serving

1. Heat the coconut oil in large skillet or wok over medium-high heat.

2. Add the garlic and ginger, and sauté for 15 seconds.

3. Add the tofu and sauté for 2 minutes.

4. Add the broccoli, bell pepper, carrot, onion, and tamari sauce. Toss and cook for 5 minutes or until the tofu is heated through and vegetables are crisp-tender.

5. Serve with brown rice.

TIP: Tamari sauce is a gluten-free alternative to soy sauce that is similar in flavor but richer in taste.

PER SERVING (WITHOUT BROWN RICE): Calories: 198; Total Fat: 10g; Saturated Fat: 4g; Carbohydrates: 15g; Fiber: 5g; Protein: 14g

STEAMED FISH AND VEGGIE PACKETS

SERVES 4; PREP TIME: 20 MINUTES
COOK TIME: 20 MINUTES

Steaming fish and vegetables in a paper packet creates a light and flavorful meal with minimal cleanup. Use any firm white fish and experiment with various veggies and herbs. The possibilities are endless.

2 cups julienned sweet potato

1 pound wild cod, cut into 4 pieces

4 tablespoons butter

8 sprigs fresh thyme

4 lemon slices

1 teaspoon kosher salt, divided

1. Preheat the oven to 425°F.

2. Fold four sheets of parchment paper in half. Place the papers on a work surface.

3. Put a pile of the sweet potato at one end of each piece of parchment paper. Top with one piece of the cod, 1 tablespoon of the butter, the thyme, and 1 slice lemon. Sprinkle ¼ teaspoon of the salt over each. Repeat with additional packets.

4. Fold the parchment paper over to form a packet and crease the edges to seal.

5. Transfer to a baking sheet and bake for 20 minutes. Let rest for 5 to 10 minutes before serving. The packets can be opened at the table.

TIP: Wild cod is a healthy choice during pregnancy because it's low in mercury. As a general rule, the smaller the fish, the less mercury it can accumulate in its lifetime.

PER SERVING: Calories: 329; Total Fat: 15g; Saturated Fat: 2g; Carbohydrates: 21g; Fiber: 2g; Protein: 28g

FISH TACOS WITH MANGO SALSA

SERVES 4; PREP TIME: 20 MINUTES
COOK TIME: 20 MINUTES

Plan a home-cooked fiesta in less than an hour. This versatile recipe is easy enough for a week-night dinner and special enough for company. The tacos are baked instead of fried, making them much lower in fat and less likely to cause heartburn.

1 pound wild cod, cut into 16 strips

1 tablespoon olive oil

Kosher salt

Freshly ground black pepper

½ cup diced red onion

1 cup diced tomato

1 cup chopped fresh mango

¼ cup fresh cilantro

8 corn tortillas, warmed

1. Preheat the oven to 400°F.

2. Line a baking sheet with parchment paper and set the fish in the pan.

3. Brush the fish with the olive oil, season with salt and pepper, and bake for 20 to 25 minutes, until cooked through.

4. In a medium bowl, combine the onion, tomato, mango, and cilantro. Mix together and set aside.

5. On 4 serving plates, fill 4 tortillas with 4 pieces of fish and top with the salsa.

6. Serve warm.

TIP: Make this recipe with grilled portobello mushrooms and black beans for a high-protein vegetarian taco.

PER SERVING: Calories: 283; Total Fat: 6g; Saturated Fat: 1g; Carbohydrates: 29g; Fiber: 4g; Protein: 29g

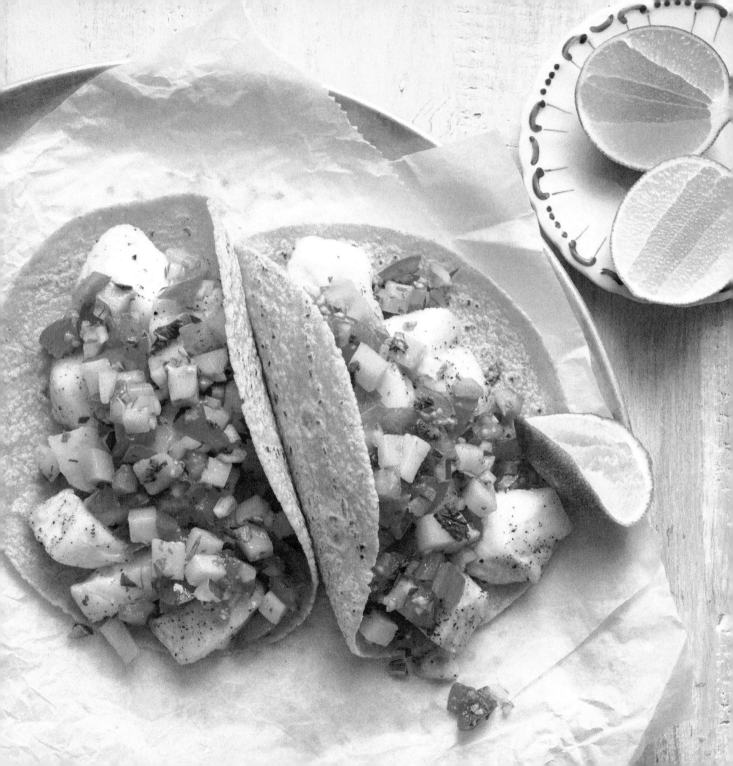

HERB ROASTED COD

**SERVES 1; PREP TIME: 15 MINUTES, PLUS
30 MINUTES TO 2 HOURS MARINATING TIME
COOK TIME: 10 MINUTES**

Cod is a mild, delicate fish that is easy to prepare and cooks quickly. A flavorful marinade turns fish into a light and elegant main course. Spices like fennel seed may help settle an upset stomach.

2 tablespoons extra-virgin olive oil

¼ cup freshly squeezed orange juice

1 teaspoon fennel seed

1 teaspoon honey

2 tablespoons chopped fresh herbs, like tarragon, thyme, parsley

½ teaspoon kosher salt

Freshly ground black pepper

6 ounces wild cod or other low-mercury white fish

1. In a large bowl, add the olive oil, orange juice, fennel seed, honey, herbs, salt, and season with pepper. Whisk together to combine.

2. Place the marinade in a deep nonreactive dish, add the fish, and let marinate for 30 minutes or up to 2 hours, turning twice to submerge all sides.

3. Preheat the broiler or a grill to high.

4. Place the fish on the grill for 5 to 7 minutes per side until cooked through.

5. Allow to rest for 5 minutes before serving.

PER SERVING: Calories: 468; Total Fat: 30g; Saturated Fat: 4g; Carbohydrates: 12g; Fiber: 11g; Protein: 39g

MANGO-SPICE CHICKEN BURGERS

**MAKES 4 BURGERS; PREP TIME: 15 MINUTES
COOK TIME: 10 MINUTES**

Ground chicken breast makes a really yummy burger and is a lean alternative. Serve on whole-wheat rolls or wrapped in lettuce cups. Make sure these poultry burgers are cooked thoroughly to an internal temperature of 165°F.

1 pound ground skinless chicken breast

½ cup chopped fresh mango

2 small scallions, chopped

¼ teaspoon ground cumin

¼ teaspoon ground turmeric

¼ teaspoon kosher salt

⅛ teaspoon freshly ground black pepper

Baby spinach, tomato, or pickles, for garnishing

1. In a large bowl, combine the chicken, mango, scallions, cumin, turmeric, salt, and pepper.

2. Mix gently with a fork and form into 4 equal burgers.

3. Grill or cook in a skillet over medium-high heat for 5 to 6 minutes per side, until cooked through.

TIP: Turmeric is a bright yellow spice with inflammation-fighting properties.

PER SERVING (WITHOUT GARNISH): Calories: 226; Total Fat: 9g; Saturated Fat: 2g; Carbohydrates: 4g; Fiber: 1g; Protein: 33g

COCONUT-CRUSTED CHICKEN STRIPS

SERVES 4; PREP TIME: 15 MINUTES
COOK TIME: 15 MINUTES

Shredded coconut gives a sweet flavor and a crunchy texture to these chicken fingers. If you're craving fried chicken but don't need the extra calories, reach for these instead. Make extra and store in the freezer in a resealable bag, then pop in the oven for a quick dinner on a busy weeknight.

2 egg whites

3 cups whole-grain cereal, crushed to crumbs in a resealable bag

¼ cup shredded unsweetened coconut

½ teaspoon kosher salt

¼ teaspoon freshly ground black pepper

1 pound boneless skinless chicken breast, cut into strips

1. Preheat the oven to 400°F.

2. Put the egg whites in a small, shallow bowl and whisk with a fork until frothy

3. Put the cereal, coconut, salt, and pepper in a food processor (or blender) and pulse to combine. Transfer the mixture to a resealable plastic bag.

4. Dredge each chicken strip in the egg white and then put in the bag. Shake the strips to coat with the coconut mixture. Place on a baking sheet and bake for 7 to 8 minutes per side, until the chicken is cooked through.

5. Serve warm.

TIP: Not a fan of coconut? These chicken fingers are just as delicious simply crusted with the crushed whole-grain cereal.

PER SERVING: Calories: 325; Total Fat: 10g; Saturated Fat: 4g; Carbohydrates: 19g; Fiber: 1g; Protein: 36g

CHICKEN QUESADILLAS

SERVES 1; PREP TIME: 15 MINUTES
COOK TIME: 10 MINUTES

Scale this recipe up for a crowd. These make a wonderful appetizer or a quick dinner that everyone will love. Experiment with different fillings, and use whatever protein, vegetables, and cheeses you have on hand.

1 tablespoon olive oil

1 (6-inch) whole-wheat flour or corn tortilla

2 ounces cooked chicken breast, sliced

¼ cup shredded Cheddar cheese

2 tablespoons sliced jalapeño chile peppers

Salsa, for serving

Sour cream, for serving

1. Heat a skillet over medium heat. Add the olive oil.

2. Lay the tortilla out flat on the work surface and put the filling in, starting with the chicken, then the cheese, and the jalapeño peppers. Fold the tortilla in half.

3. Place the folded tortilla in the skillet and cook for 3 to 4 minutes per side or until the cheese is melted and the tortilla is lightly golden.

4. Slice and serve with salsa and sour cream.

TIP: Want to make this recipe dairy free? Try with a nice-melting soy- or almond-based cheese.

PER SERVING (WITHOUT SALSA AND SOUR CREAM):
Calories: 383; Total Fat: 26g; Saturated Fat: 8g; Carbohydrates: 12g; Fiber: 2g; Protein: 27g

PERFECT ROASTED CHICKEN

SERVES 4 TO 6; PREP TIME: 15 MINUTES,
PLUS 20 MINUTES RESTING TIME
COOK TIME: 50 MINUTES

Everyone needs a go-to roast chicken recipe for entertaining and Sunday family dinners. The intoxicating aroma will fill the kitchen in minutes, making for a sensory experience before the meal even begins. Save the carcass and vegetable scraps to make chicken stock the next day.

1 (4-pound) chicken

4 rosemary sprigs

1 lemon, cut in half

2 tablespoons olive oil

Kosher salt

Freshly ground black pepper

1. Preheat the oven to 400°F.

2. Place the chicken in a 12-inch cast-iron skillet or roasting pan.

3. Place the rosemary sprigs and lemon halves in the cavity.

4. Rub the chicken all over with the olive oil and season with salt and pepper.

5. Roast for 50 to 60 minutes or until internal temperature reaches 165°F.

6. Allow to rest for at least 20 minutes before slicing.

7. Serve warm with a vegetable and salad for a complete meal.

PER SERVING: Calories: 336; Total Fat: 8g; Saturated Fat: 2g; Carbohydrates: 1g; Fiber: 0g; Protein: 66g

SLOW COOKER BALSAMIC CHICKEN

SERVES 4; PREP TIME: 10 MINUTES
COOK TIME: 6 HOURS

Every new mom needs a few simple set-it-and-forget-it recipes. Toss the ingredients in and let the slow cooker do the work. Chicken thighs are healthier than most people think: they are packed with flavor and heart-healthy unsaturated fats.

1 cup sliced onions

2 cups sliced bell peppers

1 cup diced tomato

1 pound boneless, skinless chicken thighs

2 tablespoons balsamic vinegar

½ teaspoon kosher salt

1. Preheat a slow cooker on low.

2. Put the vegetables in the bottom of the cooker. Put the chicken pieces on top and sprinkle with the vinegar and salt.

3. Cover and cook for 6 hours.

4. Remove the chicken and vegetables to a platter. Shred the chicken with two forks before serving, if desired.

TIP: Experiment with different kinds of vegetables in this recipe, like string beans and broccoli. Add them to the pot during the last 20 minutes of cooking to keep them crisp-tender and to retain their nutrient content.

PER SERVING: Calories: 181; Total Fat 5g; Saturated Fat: 1g; Carbohydrates: 10; Fiber: 2g; Protein: 25g

CHICKEN-QUINOA STUFFED PEPPERS

SERVES 6; PREP TIME: 15 MINUTES
COOK TIME: 40 MINUTES

Stuffed pepper recipes are often considered "old school," but this version has all kinds of new twists and offers the nutrients you need to help support healthy growth and development. Quinoa, beans, chicken, mushrooms, and a touch of cheese come together in a delicious edible package.

6 red bell peppers

1 tablespoon olive oil

6 ounces cooked chicken

2 cups sliced mushrooms

¼ cup finely chopped red onion

½ teaspoon kosher salt

¼ teaspoon black pepper

1 cup canned black beans, drained and rinsed

1 garlic clove, minced

1 cup salsa

1½ cups cooked quinoa

½ cup shredded mozzarella cheese

1. Preheat the oven to 350°F.

2. Cut off the tops of the bell peppers and scoop out the seeds. Set aside.

3. Heat the olive oil in a large skillet over medium-high heat. Add the chicken, mushrooms, onion, salt, and pepper, and sauté for about 5 minutes or until tender.

4. Add the beans, garlic, and salsa, and sauté for 2 minutes. Turn off the heat and mix in the quinoa. Fill each bell pepper with the quinoa mixture and top with the shredded cheese.

5. Transfer the bell peppers to a baking dish, cover with aluminum foil, and bake for 15 minutes. Remove the foil and bake for 15 minutes more.

6. Allow to cool for 10 minutes before serving.

PER SERVING: Calories: 276; Total Fat: 7g; Saturated Fat: 2g; Carbohydrates: 33g; Fiber: 8g; Protein: 20g

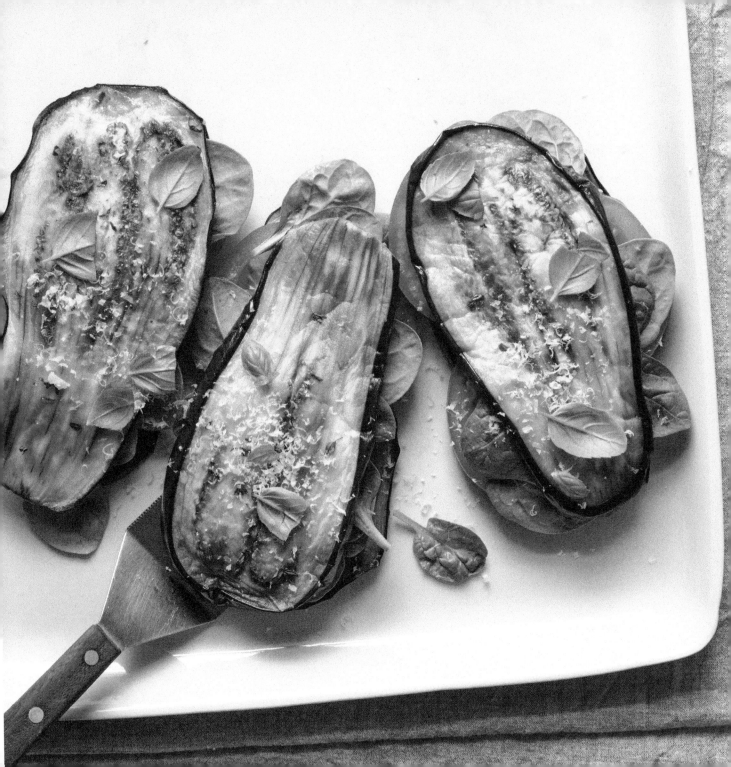

EGGPLANT STACKERS

SERVES 6; PREP TIME: 20 MINUTES
COOK TIME: 15 MINUTES

These stackers are sandwiches with thin slices of roasted eggplant as the bread. The eggplant can be prepared ahead of time. Substitute the fillings depending on what fresh vegetables are in season. The eggplant can be replaced with zucchini or butternut squash.

1 large eggplant, cut crosswise into 12 thin slices

2 tablespoons olive oil

Kosher salt

Dried thyme

1 tomato, cut into 6 slices

2 cups baby spinach

Toppings: Marinara Sauce (page 182), Parmesan cheese, or balsamic vinaigrette

1. Preheat the oven to 400°F.

2. Place the eggplant slices in a sheet pan. Brush with the olive oil and season with salt and thyme.

3. Bake for 15 to 20 minutes until tender.

4. To assemble start with an eggplant slice followed by a tomato slice and a pile of spinach. End with a second eggplant slice. Repeat to make five more stackers.

5. Serve with the toppings of your choice.

PER SERVING (WITHOUT TOPPING): Calories: 200; Total Fat: 14g; Saturated Fat: 2g; Carbohydrates: 16g; Fiber: 8g; Protein: 3g

CAST-IRON SLIDERS

SERVES 6; PREP TIME: 15 MINUTES
COOK TIME: 10 MINUTES

You might never use an outdoor grill again after making these tiny burgers. Cast-iron skillets are easy to use and clean, plus cooking with them actually imparts iron into the food you're cooking.

1 pound ground turkey

Kosher salt

Freshly ground black pepper

6 small whole-grain rolls, sliced in half

1. Divide the turkey into 6 equal balls.

2. Heat a cast-iron skillet over medium-high heat.

3. Place 3 turkey balls in the skillet and press them with a spatula to flatten slightly.

4. Season with salt and pepper.

5. Cook for 2 to 3 minutes, then flip and cook 2 to 3 minutes on the other side. Repeat for the other 3 turkey balls.

6. Toast the rolls cut-side down in the skillet until golden.

7. Serve the sliders hot.

PER SERVING: Calories: 238; Total Fat: 9g; Saturated Fat: 2g; Carbohydrates: 24g; Fiber: 4g; Protein: 18g

TACO SALAD CUPS

SERVES 4; PREP TIME: 5 MINUTES
COOK TIME: 10 MINUTES

Feeling like having a fiesta? Make these lettuce cups for a winning Mexican dinner. Replace the meat with chopped cooked mushrooms for a vegetarian version. And if you've been suffering from heartburn, skip the chili powder and go easy on the beans.

2 teaspoons olive oil

½ cup chopped red onion

½ cup diced bell pepper

½ teaspoon kosher salt

1 garlic clove, minced

1 pound ground turkey breast

½ teaspoon ground cumin

½ teaspoon chili powder

1 cup canned black beans, drained and rinsed

1 head large-leaf lettuce, such as Bibb or iceberg, for cups

¼ cup shredded lowfat Cheddar cheese

1. Heat the oil in a large skillet over medium-high heat Add the onion, bell pepper, and salt, and sauté for 3 minutes.

2. Add the garlic and turkey, and sauté until meat is browned, about 5 minutes.

3. Add the cumin, chili powder, and black beans, and stir well to combine. Cook for 2 minutes until heated through.

4. Serve in the lettuce cups topped with the cheese.

PER SERVING: Calories: 374; Total Fat: 12g; Saturated Fat: 4g; Carbohydrates: 20g; Fiber: 5g; Protein: 39g

BAKED MEATBALLS

MAKES 16 MEATBALLS; PREP TIME: 15 MINUTES
COOK TIME: 25 MINUTES

Need more iron in your diet? Make moist and delicious lowfat meatballs. Baking them is the easy way to go, and they're ready to eat in less than 30 minutes. Serve along with a green salad or with your favorite whole-grain pasta and tomato sauce.

1 pound lean ground turkey (93% lean)

1 large egg, beaten

4 tablespoons ground almonds

1 garlic clove, minced

1 tablespoon chopped fresh basil

1 teaspoon kosher salt

½ teaspoon freshly ground black pepper

1. Preheat oven to 400°F. Line a baking sheet with parchment paper.

2. In a large bowl, combine the ground turkey, egg, almonds, garlic, basil, salt, and pepper. Gently combine the mixture well and form into sixteen 1-ounce balls.

3. Transfer to the prepared baking sheet. Bake for 20 minutes or until internal temperature reaches 165°F. Serve hot.

PER MEATBALL: Calories: 54; Total Fat: 3g; Saturated Fat: 1g; Carbohydrates: 1g; Fiber: 0g; Protein: 6g

STUFFED SWEET POTATO BAR

SERVES 4; PREP TIME: 5 MINUTES
COOK TIME: NONE

Set up a stuffed sweet potato bar for dinner one night this week. Bake potatoes ahead of time so all you have to do is prepare the fixings. Sweet potatoes are rich in beta-carotene, the plant-based form of vitamin A that is so important for healthy skin and good eyesight.

4 baked sweet potatoes

16 ounces cooked tofu or beans

4 cups cooked vegetables, like spinach, kale, broccoli, mushrooms

¼ cup lowfat Greek yogurt

Cut the sweet potatoes in half and top with the tofu, vegetables, and a dollop of Greek yogurt.

PER SERVING (WITH TOFU): Calories: 263; Total Fat: 7g; Saturated Fat: 1g; Carbohydrates: 34g; Fiber: 10g; Protein: 20g

PARSLEY PESTO PASTA

**SERVES 6; PREP TIME: 15 MINUTES
COOK TIME: 10 MINUTES**

This mild pesto adds flavor and a splash of green to marinades, salad dressings, and pasta. Fresh herbs are an underappreciated source of nutrition. They are filled with vitamins A, C, and K, as well as various antioxidants; they are also a fabulous ingredient to boost flavor without a lot of extra calories.

4 cups fresh parsley

1 garlic clove, chopped

Juice and zest of 1 lemon

¼ cup grated Parmesan cheese (optional)

1 teaspoon kosher salt

½ teaspoon freshly ground black pepper

¾ cup extra-virgin olive oil

1 pound whole-grain pasta

1. To make the parsley pesto, in a food processor (or blender) fitted with a steel blade, combine the parsley, garlic, lemon juice and zest, Parmesan cheese (omit the Parmesan from the recipe if you will be freezing the extra pesto), salt, and pepper.

2. Pulse until smooth. With the machine running, slowly pour in the olive oil and blend until smooth.

3. Cook the pasta according to package directions. Drain.

4. Toss the pesto with the pasta.

5. Serve warm or at room temperature.

6. To freeze the extra pesto, pour the pesto in a quart-size resealable plastic bag. Lay it flat in the freezer until it is frozen solid. You can break off pieces of the frozen pesto as needed and reseal the bag. It will keep in the freezer for up to 3 months.

TIP: Whole-grain pasta provides fiber, helping to make this pasta dish very satisfying. To round out the meal, add white beans to the pasta or serve with a side salad that includes chickpeas.

PER SERVING (WITHOUT PARMESAN CHEESE):
Calories: 525; Total Fat: 29g; Saturated Fat: 4g; Carbohydrates: 57g; Fiber: 8g; Protein: 12g

EVERYDAY SPAGHETTI

**SERVES 6; PREP TIME: 15 MINUTES
COOK TIME: 25 MINUTES**

You will most likely crave this classic comfort food at some point in your pregnancy. This recipe makes it wonderfully easy. For a freezer meal, instead of spaghetti, mix the sauce with cooked ziti in a casserole dish and top with cheese. Seal the dish with plastic wrap and foil, and store in the freezer for a homemade dinner after the baby arrives.

1 tablespoon olive oil

1 garlic clove, minced

¼ cup chopped red onion

3 cups diced canned tomatoes

1 teaspoon kosher salt

½ cup fresh basil leaves, chopped

Baked Meatballs (page 175)

1 pound whole-grain spaghetti

1. Heat the olive oil in a medium saucepan over medium heat. Add the garlic and onion, and sauté, stirring, for 5 minutes.

2. Add the tomatoes, salt, and basil, and stir to combine. Simmer for 20 minutes. Remove from the heat. Purée with an immersion blender (or countertop blender) and keep warm.

3. Cook the spaghetti according to the package directions. Drain.

4. Serve the spaghetti topped with tomato sauce and baked turkey meatballs.

PER SERVING: Calories: 447; Total Fat: 11g; Saturated Fat: 4g; Carbohydrates: 61g; Fiber: 3g; Protein: 24g

GRILLED TOMATO BASIL PIZZA

SERVES 4; PREP TIME: 5 MINUTES
COOK TIME: 10 MINUTES

Make homemade pizza a tradition for your growing family. With so many ways to prepare it, you can experiment with different flavors and toppings as your child grows. Cooking raw tomatoes also boosts the lycopene, an important cell-protecting antioxidant. For extra flavor, drizzle the cooked pizza with a fruity extra-virgin olive oil.

12 ounces store-bought refrigerated ready-made pizza dough

1 tomato, sliced

8 ounces fresh goat cheese

8 fresh basil leaves

½ cup grated Parmesan cheese

1. Heat the grill to medium-high.

2. Roll out the pizza dough into a 12-inch circle (it doesn't have to be perfect).

3. Place on the grill and cook for 2 minutes, watching carefully to be sure the crust doesn't burn.

4. Using tongs, flip the pizza dough over.

5. Top the cooked side with the sliced tomatoes and goat cheese.

6. Cook for 5 to 8 minutes or until the goat cheese is melted.

7. Remove from the grill and top with torn basil leaves and Parmesan cheese.

TIP: Instead of grilling the pizza, you can bake it in a 450-degree oven.

PER SERVING: Calories: 400; Total Fat: 19g; Saturated Fat: 10g; Carbohydrates: 42g; Fiber: 2g; Protein: 18g

ROASTED TOFU RICE BOWLS

**SERVES 4; PREP TIME: 20 MINUTES
COOK TIME: 20 MINUTES**

Don't think you like tofu? Then you haven't tried this recipe yet. When combined with rice and vegetables, this meal is beyond satisfying.

1 package extra-firm tofu

2 tablespoons olive oil

1 teaspoon honey

4 cups cooked brown rice

1 cup cooked peeled edamame

1 cup shredded carrots

½ cup chopped cashews

2 tablespoons chopped fresh cilantro

1. Dice the tofu block into cubes and drain on a paper towel for 10 minutes to remove excess water.

2. Preheat the oven to 425°F.

3. In a large bowl, whisk the olive oil and honey together.

4. Add the tofu and gently toss to coat. Transfer to a sheet pan and bake for 20 to 25 minutes, turning once, until golden brown.

5. Assemble 4 bowls with rice, tofu, edamame, carrots, and cashews.

6. Top with the fresh cilantro and serve.

PER SERVING: Calories: 428; Total Fat: 18g; Saturated Fat: 3g; Carbohydrates: 50g; Fiber: 5g; Protein: 16g

VEGETABLE FRIED RICE

SERVES 4; PREP TIME: 10 MINUTES
COOK TIME: 15 MINUTES

You won't miss the meat in this savory and satisfying dish. It is also excellent when made with leftover chicken or tofu. When making rice, make extra to have on hand for this dish. Use leftover protein and whatever vegetables are in the kitchen.

2 teaspoons toasted sesame oil

¼ cup low-sodium tamari sauce

2 tablespoons rice vinegar

2 tablespoons olive oil, divided

1 large egg, beaten

2 cups chopped fresh green beans

1 cup grated carrot

1 cup chopped mushrooms

4 cups cooked brown rice

1. In a small bowl, whisk together the sesame oil, tamari sauce, and rice vinegar. Set aside.

2. Heat 1 tablespoon of the olive oil in a large wok or skillet over medium-high heat. Add the egg and gently scramble. Remove from the pan and set aside.

3. Heat the remaining 1 tablespoon olive oil in the wok. Add the green beans, carrot, and mushrooms, and sauté for 2 to 3 minutes.

4. Add the sauce mixture and sauté for 2 minutes.

5. Add the rice and egg, and continue cooking, stirring frequently, until all ingredients are heated through, about 5 minutes.

TIP: For some extra crunch and omega-3 fats, top with chopped walnuts.

PER SERVING: Calories: 490; Total Fat: 13g; Saturated Fat: 2g; Carbohydrates: 81g; Fiber: 6g; Protein: 12g

WHEAT BERRY AND QUINOA BURGERS

**MAKES 6 BURGERS; PREP TIME: 15 MINUTES
COOK TIME: 20 MINUTES**

You can make a darn tasty burger without any meat in sight. These whole-grain delights are packed with tummy-pleasing fiber, protein, and flavor. They have a hearty texture and nutty taste, and are filled with energy-producing B vitamins to support metabolism. Serve on buns with salad garnishes, if desired.

3 teaspoons olive oil, divided

2 tablespoons chopped white onion

1 cup cooked wheat berries, cooled

1 cup cooked quinoa

¼ cup finely diced red bell pepper

2 tablespoons hummus

1 large egg

¼ teaspoon kosher salt

¼ teaspoon freshly ground black pepper

1. In a food processor (or blender), combine 1 teaspoon of olive oil, the onion, wheat berries, quinoa, bell pepper, hummus, egg, salt, and black pepper.

2. Pulse until the mixture is well combined.

3. Form the mixture into 6 equal patties, using about ½ cup for each.

4. Heat the remaining 2 teaspoons of olive oil in a large skillet over medium-high heat. Put 2 to 3 burgers in the skillet and cook for 5 minutes per side. Transfer to a plate and cook the remaining burgers.

5. Serve hot.

TIP: To cook the whole grains like wheat berries and quinoa, place 1 cup of dry grains in a pot with 2 cups of water and a pinch of salt (always use double the measure of water to dry grains). Bring to a boil, reduce to a simmer, cover, and cook until the grains are tender and the water is absorbed. Cooking times vary. Quinoa will take about 15 minutes. Let cool before using.

PER SERVING: Calories: 176; Total Fat: 8g; Saturated Fat: 1g; Carbohydrates: 23g; Fiber: 5g; Protein: 7g

ZOODLES MARINARA

**SERVES 4; PREP TIME: 20 MINUTES
COOK TIME: 30 MINUTES**

Spiralized veggies are a healthy and fun way to get more vitamins into your diet. Summer squash, like zucchini, is high in vitamins A, C, K, and folate—vital nutrients for healthy skin, nerves, and blood cells. A serving of protein makes a complete meal.

For the Marinara Sauce

1 tablespoon olive oil

¼ cup chopped white onion

1 garlic clove, chopped

1 (28-ounce) can crushed tomatoes

1 teaspoon kosher salt

½ cup chopped fresh basil

For the Zoodles

3 large summer squash, such as zucchini or yellow crookneck, unpeeled

1 tablespoon extra-virgin olive oil

½ teaspoon kosher salt

Chopped fresh basil and shredded Parmesan cheese, for serving

To Make the Marinara Sauce

1. Heat the olive oil in a medium saucepan over medium-high heat.

2. Add the onion and garlic and sauté until onion is translucent, about 10 minutes.

3. Stir in the tomatoes and salt, and simmer, stirring often, for 20 minutes.

4. Stir in the basil and serve immediately on the zoodles.

5. The sauce can be stored in the refrigerator for up to 1 week or frozen for up to 3 months.

To Make the Zoodles

1. Cut the squash into spirals or strips using a spiralizer tool (see Tip below).

2. Heat the olive oil in a large skillet over medium-high heat. Add the squash and salt, and cook, stirring frequently, for 2 to 3 minutes.

3. Add the marinara sauce and continue to cook until the zoodles are slightly wilted, about 5 minutes.

4. Serve sprinkled with fresh basil.

TIP: Several kitchen tools in many price ranges that can create "zoodles," or long strands of vegetables.

PER SERVING: Calories: 138; Total Fat: 6g; Saturated Fat: 1g; Carbohydrates: 6g; Fiber: 4g; Protein: 6g

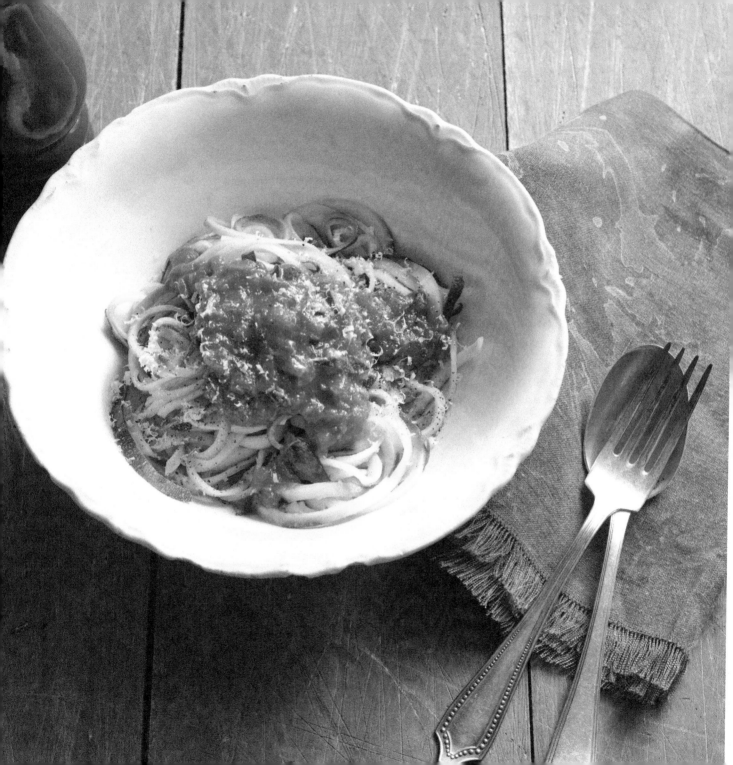

SPAGHETTI SQUASH PARMESAN

SERVES 2; PREP TIME: 5 MINUTES
COOK TIME: 25 MINUTES

This squash doesn't exactly taste like pasta, but for a lower-carb alternative it really works! Roasting in the oven makes it very tender and enhances the natural sweetness of the squash. Top with marinara sauce and cheese, and you create a satisfying vegetarian and gluten-free meal.

1 spaghetti squash

2 tablespoons olive oil

Kosher salt

Freshly ground black pepper

½ cup Marinara Sauce (see page 182)

½ cup shredded mozzarella cheese

1. Preheat the oven to 400°F.

2. Line a sheet pan with aluminum foil.

3. Cut the squash in half lengthwise and scoop out the seeds.

4. Season the cut side with olive oil, salt, and pepper.

5. Place the halves cut-side down on the baking sheet, and bake for 20 to 25 minutes or until fork-tender.

6. Turn over and top the cut side with sauce and sprinkle with cheese.

7. Return to the oven and bake for 5 minutes or until the cheese is melted and bubbling.

PER SERVING: Calories: 280; Total Fat: 21g; Saturated Fat: 5g; Carbohydrates: 16g; Fiber: 4g; Protein: 9g

ONE-SIZE-FITS-ALL MARINADE

MAKES ABOUT ⅔ CUP; PREP TIME: 5 MINUTES, PLUS 2 HOURS MARINATING TIME COOK TIME: VARIES

This marinade tastes good on just about everything. It's sweet, savory, and tangy to excite your senses and satisfy your cravings. Vegetables, chicken thighs, and salmon are some of the tastiest options.

½ cup reduced-sodium tamari sauce

¼ cup rice vinegar

2 tablespoons raw honey

1 garlic clove, minced

1. Whisk all the ingredients together in a small bowl.

2. To prepare, marinate for 2 hours (chicken can go for up to 24 hours), then grill or broil.

3. Store in an airtight glass container in the refrigerator for up to 1 week.

PER SERVING (1 TABLESPOON): Calories: 22; Total Fat: 0g; Saturated Fat: 0g; Carbohydrates: 4g; Fiber: 0g; Protein: 1g

VEGGIE KEBAB

SERVES 4; PREP TIME: 15 MINUTES COOK TIME: 10 MINUTES

For some reason, food on a stick just tastes better. Here's a fun way to get more vegetables in, plus get a large amount of antioxidants to help fight inflammation.

1 small red bell pepper, cut into chunks

1 small green bell pepper, cut into chunks

1 small zucchini or yellow squash, cut into 1-inch rounds

1 package (12 ounces) whole mushrooms, cleaned and stems trimmed

1 tablespoon olive oil

Juice of 1 lime

¼ teaspoon kosher salt

¼ teaspoon freshly ground black pepper

1. Preheat the grill to medium heat.

2. Slide vegetables onto 4 metal or wooden skewers, alternating the bell peppers, zucchini, and mushrooms.

3. In a small bowl, whisk together the olive oil, lime juice, salt, and pepper.

4. Brush the mixture onto the skewered vegetables.

5. Grill on medium heat for 10 to 15 minutes, until the vegetables are warm and slightly tender.

PER SERVING: Calories: 45; Total Fat: 1.5g; Saturated Fat: 0g; Carbohydrates: 6g; Fiber: 2g; Protein: 1g

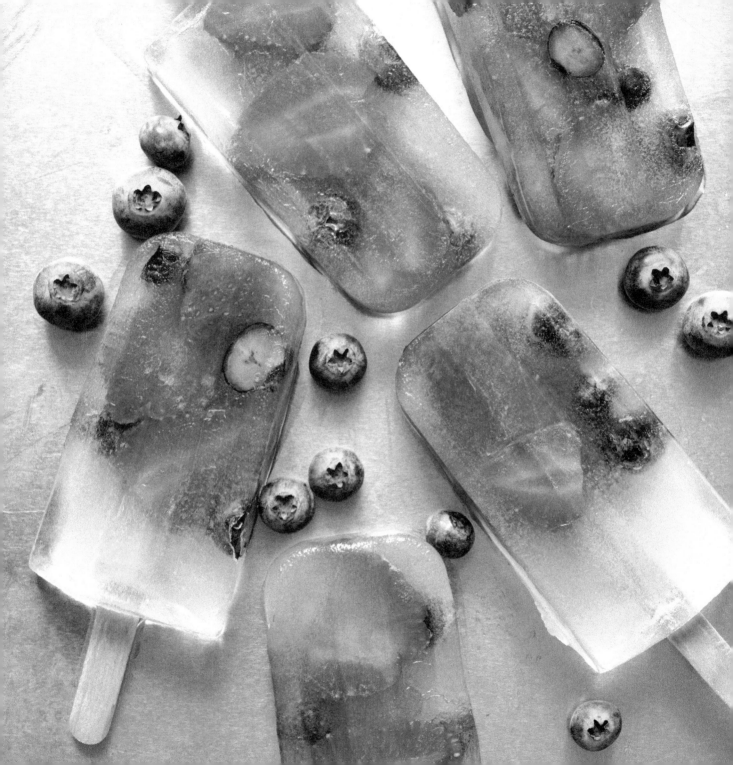

twelve

DESSERTS

....

STRAWBERRY GRANITA

SERVES 4; PREP TIME: 5 MINUTES,
PLUS 4 HOURS FREEZING TIME
COOK TIME: 5 MINUTES

Pass on the fast-food slushie drinks and make this sweet, icy treat with real fruit! It's a cool dessert to help you beat the heat on a hot summer day, plus it will help keep you hydrated.

1 pint strawberries, washed and hulled

4 cups brewed decaf green tea

1. Combine the berries and tea in a medium saucepan. Bring to a boil, reduce heat to medium, and cook for 5 to 7 minutes.

2. Strain the mixture through a fine-mesh strainer, using a rubber spatula to press the juices through.

3. Transfer the liquid to a shallow glass baking dish and place in the freezer.

4. Once the mixture begins to freeze, about 1 hour, scrape with a fork to create ice crystals every 30 minutes until the mixture is completely frozen.

5. Scoop ice shavings into 4 small bowls and serve immediately.

PER SERVING: Calories: 39; Total Fat 0g; Saturated Fat: 0g; Carbohydrates: 9g; Fiber: 2g; Protein: 1g

CHAMOMILE BERRY ICE POPS

SERVES 4; PREP TIME: 5 MINUTES,
PLUS 3 HOURS FREEZING TIME
COOK TIME: NONE

You can make an ice pop out of just about anything. Pour leftover brewed tea into a popsicle mold and add fresh fruit. It's such a flavorful way to stay hydrated. Chamomile tea also helps you relax after an exhausting day on your feet.

3 cups cool chamomile tea

Fresh berries, such as raspberries, blackberries, or sliced strawberries

1. Pour the tea into popsicle molds.

2. Add a few berries into each mold.

3. Put molds in freezer until frozen solid, about 3 hours.

PER SERVING: Calories: 20; Total Fat: 0g; Saturated Fat: 0g; Carbohydrates: 6g; Fiber: 2g; Protein: 0g

COCONUT-LIME
ICE POPS

SERVES 4; PREP TIME: 5 MINUTES,
PLUS 3 HOURS FREEZING TIME
COOK TIME: NONE

Cool and creamy, coconut milk makes the most delicious frozen desserts. If you're craving a tropical cocktail, make these and pretend you are on vacation instead of at home with swollen ankles.

1 (14-ounce) can full-fat coconut milk

Zest of 1 lime

1. Combine the coconut milk and lime zest in a small bowl and whisk together well.

2. Pour the mixture into 4 popsicle molds.

3. Put in the freezer until frozen solid, about 3 hours.

TIP: Coconut milk is super-sweet and doesn't require extra sweeteners when used in a recipe.

PER SERVING: Calories: 165; Total Fat: 18g; Saturated Fat: 16g; Carbohydrates: 2g; Fiber: 0g; Protein: 2g

FROZEN
BANANA POPS

SERVES 4; PREP TIME: 5 MINUTES,
PLUS 1 HOUR FREEZING TIME
COOK TIME: NONE

Here's a frozen treat without having to chase down the ice-cream truck. If you're craving ice cream and chocolate, make these pops and keep them on hand in the freezer. Wrapped in plastic, they will keep for up to 1 month. Choose a dark chocolate that's 80% cacao.

2 bananas, cut in half

½ cup dark chocolate chips, melted in a shallow dish

Chopped nuts, in a shallow dish

4 popsicle sticks

1. Dip each banana half into the melted chocolate, then roll in the nuts.

2. Place the bananas on a plate or small sheet pan and insert a popsicle stick into each banana from the end.

3. Freeze for about 1 hour or until the chocolate has hardened.

PER SERVING: Calories: 180; Total Fat: 9g; Saturated Fat: 4g; Carbohydrates: 28g; Fiber: 3g; Protein: 2g

ONE-INGREDIENT ICE CREAM

SERVES 4; PREP TIME: 5 MINUTES
COOK TIME: NONE

You may not believe that frozen fruit could take the place of creamy ice cream, but this recipe will change your mind! When you have that large bunch of bananas on the counter that are about to go bad, store them in the freezer for smoothies and for this dairy-free ice cream alternative.

8 bananas, chopped and frozen

1. Place frozen bananas in a food processor (or blender) and pulse until the mixture is smooth and creamy (similar to soft serve ice cream).

2. Serve immediately, or for a harder consistency, place the mixture in the freezer for 1 hour to harden.

TIP: Adding goodies like cocoa powder, fresh fruit, and nuts makes this ice cream even better. You can refreeze this mixture. It will get a little icy but still taste delicious.

PER SERVING: Calories: 210; Total Fat: 1g; Saturated Fat: 0g; Carbohydrates: 54g; Fiber: 6g; Protein: 3g

FROZEN YOGURT PARFAIT

SERVES 4; PREP TIME: 5 MINUTES,
PLUS ICE-CREAM MACHINE TIME
COOK TIME: NONE

A quick spin in the ice-cream machine and you can create a much lower fat and higher protein version of your favorite soft serve from yogurt. Add any kind of fruit preserves or fresh fruit to the mixture.

3 cups lowfat vanilla Greek yogurt
2 tablespoons fruit preserves
Mint leaves, for garnish (optional)

1. In a large bowl, whisk the yogurt and preserves together.

2. Place in an ice-cream machine and prepare according to the manufacturer's directions.

3. Chill 4 parfait glasses and fill them with the frozen yogurt. Garnish with mint leaves (if using).

TIP: Greek yogurt is lower in lactose and is often tolerated better than regular yogurt by those with lactose intolerance.

PER SERVING: Calories: 137; Total Fat: 3g; Saturated Fat: 2g; Carbohydrates: 13g; Fiber: 0g; Protein: 14g

COCOA MILKSHAKE

SERVES 1; PREP TIME: 5 MINUTES
COOK TIME: NONE

A small amount of chocolate decadence goes a very long way in this milkshake. Bananas and lowfat milk combine with ice to create a slimmer version of a creamy milkshake. This recipe can easily be made dairy-free by using coconut, almond, or soy milk.

2 bananas

1 tablespoon unsweetened cocoa powder

1 cup lowfat milk or nondairy milk alternative

4 ice cubes

1. Combine the banana, cocoa, milk, and ice in a blender and blend until smooth.

2. Pour into a tall glass and serve with a straw.

PER SERVING: Calories: 342; Total Fat: 4g; Saturated Fat: 1g; Carbohydrates: 82g; Fiber: 8g; Protein: 4g

AVOCADO ICE CREAM

SERVES 4; PREP TIME: 5 MINUTES,
PLUS ICE-CREAM MACHINE TIME
AND 1 HOUR FREEZING TIME
COOK TIME: NONE

Did you know that avocado is actually a fruit? The vibrant green flesh is high in heart-healthy fats and has a wonderful texture, making it an ideal base for a frozen dessert. This recipe isn't only dairy-free, it's vegan because it contains no animal products.

2 avocados, flesh scooped out

Juice of ½ lemon

2 (14-ounce) cans unsweetened full-fat coconut milk

¼ cup raw honey

1. Place the ingredients in a blender and blend until smooth.

2. Transfer the mixture to an ice cream machine and prepare according to the manufacturer's suggestions.

3. Transfer to an airtight container and put it in the freezer to harden for at least 1 hour.

PER SERVING: Calories: 564; Total Fat: 52g; Saturated Fat: 39g; Carbohydrates: 29g; Fiber: 5g; Protein: 5g

PEACH-BLUEBERRY CRISP

SERVES 6; PREP TIME: 10 MINUTES
COOK TIME: 30 MINUTES

Fruit crisps are one of the healthiest and easiest desserts to make. Use any kind of seasonal fruit, or use frozen fruit, which is actually as nutritious as fresh and often more affordable. Serve this version warm from the oven with a dollop of Greek yogurt on top.

4 cups blueberries

2 large peaches, peeled and diced

Juice of ½ lemon

2 tablespoons pure maple syrup

2 tablespoons coconut oil

2 tablespoons whole-wheat flour

½ cup rolled oats

½ teaspoon kosher salt

Pinch ground cinnamon

⅓ cup sliced almonds

1. Preheat the oven to 350°F.

2. In a large bowl, combine the blueberries, peaches, lemon juice, and maple syrup. Mix and set aside for 10 minutes.

3. In a separate medium bowl, combine the coconut oil, flour, oats, salt, cinnamon, and almonds.

4. Pour the fruit mixture into a 1½-quart baking dish and sprinkle evenly with the oats mixture.

5. Bake for 30 minutes or until golden and bubbly.

6. Let cool for 10 to 15 minutes before serving.

PER SERVING: Calories: 187; Total Fat: 8g; Saturated Fat: 4g; Carbohydrates: 29g; Fiber: 4g; Protein: 3g

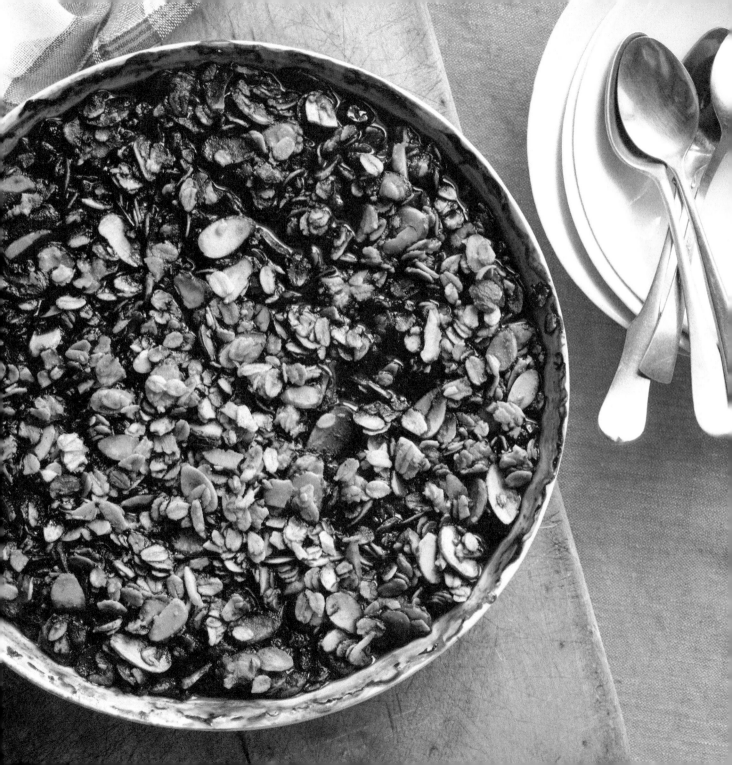

STRAWBERRIES WITH ALMOND BUTTER

SERVES 2; PREP TIME: 5 MINUTES
COOK TIME: NONE

A wonderful balance of healthy and decadent, a few spoonfuls of almond butter turns fresh fruit into dessert. Flavor the almond butter with low-calorie seasonings such as ground cinnamon, unsweetened cocoa powder, or orange zest.

¼ cup Homemade Almond Butter (page 124)

2 cups fresh strawberries, rinsed and blotted dry with a towel

1. Place the almond butter in a small shallow dish.

2. Put the strawberries in a medium serving bowl and dip them into the almond butter.

PER SERVING: Calories: 241; Total Fat: 18g; Saturated Fat: 2g; Carbohydrates: 18g; Fiber: 6g; Protein: 8g

DARK CHOCOLATE-DIPPED ORANGES

SERVES: 1; PREP TIME: 5 MINUTES
COOK TIME: 30 SECONDS

Dark chocolate is higher in antioxidants and slightly lower in fat, but that doesn't make it a health food. It still needs to be consumed in moderation. Pair chocolate with a high-fiber fruit like oranges to help make it more filling.

1 orange, peeled and segmented

1 ounce dark chocolate, melted in a small shallow bowl

Coarse sea salt (optional)

1. Dip the orange segments into melted chocolate and sprinkle with sea salt, if desired.

2. Eat them warm or place them in the freezer for 5 minutes to help set the chocolate.

TIP: You can melt the chocolate in a glass bowl in the microwave. It takes only about 30 seconds.

PER SERVING: Calories: 238; Total Fat: 9g; Saturated Fat: 6g; Carbohydrates: 39g; Fiber: 6g; Protein: 4g

FLOURLESS PEANUT BUTTER COOKIES

MAKES 24 COOKIES; PREP TIME: 10 MINUTES
COOK TIME: 10 MINUTES

These gluten-free cookies are the ultimate for any peanut butter lover. You can also add chocolate chips if you prefer the winning combo of peanut butter and chocolate. All varieties of peanut butter work well in this recipe, so use whatever you've got on hand.

1 cup peanut butter

1 cup cooked chickpeas, puréed

1 egg, lightly beaten

¼ cup finely chopped pitted dates

1 tablespoon sesame seeds

1 teaspoon pure vanilla extract

1. Preheat the oven to 350°F.

2. Line a baking sheet with parchment paper.

3. Combine all the ingredients in a medium bowl and mix until well combined.

4. Using a tablespoon or mini ice cream scoop, drop 12 equal dollops of dough onto the prepared baking sheet.

5. Bake for 8 to 10 minutes until golden. Repeat with the remaining dough.

TIP: You can freeze balls of the cookie dough on a parchment paper–lined baking sheet. Once frozen, transfer them to a resealable plastic bag. When ready to bake, place the frozen cookie dough balls onto a lined baking sheet and increase the baking time by 2 to 3 minutes.

PER COOKIE: Calories: 88; Total Fat: 6g; Saturated Fat: 1g; Carbohydrates: 5g; Fiber: 2g; Protein: 3g

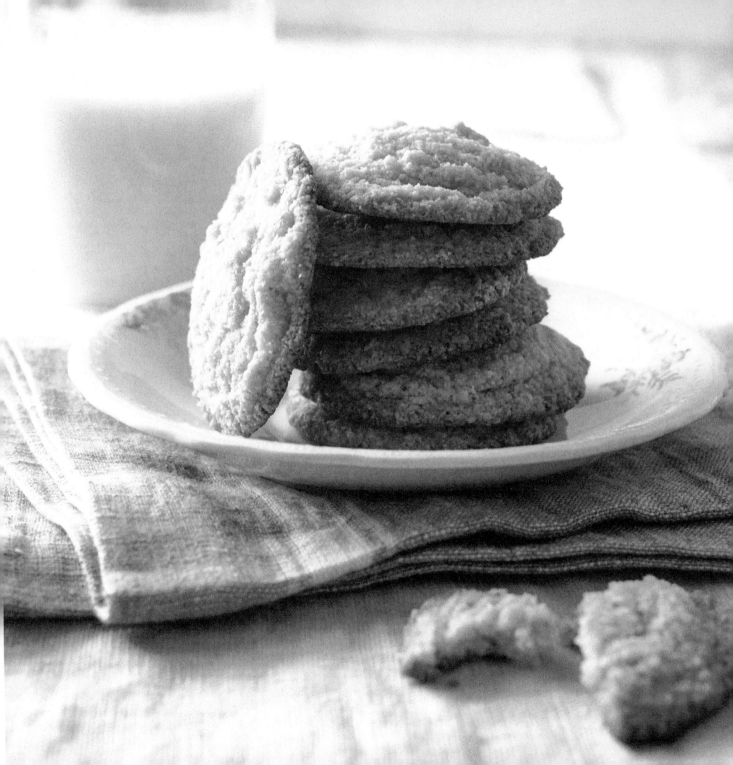

ALMOND COOKIES

MAKES 16 COOKIES; PREP TIME: 10 MINUTES
COOK TIME: 10 MINUTES

These crunchy, nutty cookies taste decadent, but almond flour makes then gluten-free and rich in nutrients. When chocolate cravings strike, add a small handful of dark chocolate chips to the batter.

1¾ cups almond flour

¼ teaspoon baking soda

¼ teaspoon kosher salt

3 tablespoons melted coconut oil

¼ cup pure maple syrup

¼ cup applesauce

1. Preheat the oven to 350°F. Line a baking sheet with parchment paper.

2. In a small bowl, whisk together the almond flour, baking soda, and salt. Set aside.

3. In a separate small bowl, combine the coconut oil, maple syrup, and applesauce.

4. Add the flour mixture to the applesauce mixture and stir well until a dough is formed.

5. Drop spoonfuls of dough onto the prepared baking sheet. Bake for 7 to 10 minutes until golden brown. Store in an airtight container at room temperature for up to 3 days.

PER COOKIE: Calories: 84; Total Fat: 8g; Saturated Fat: 3g; Carbohydrates: 3g; Fiber: 1g; Protein: 2g

GRILLED PINEAPPLE

SERVES 4; PREP TIME: 5 MINUTES
COOK TIME: 5 MINUTES

Grilling pineapple enhances the natural sweetness, making it taste more like candy! Pineapple also contains an enzyme called bromelain that is known to fight bloating and inflammation. You can use an outdoor grill but an indoor grill pan works even better. Serve with a dollop of Greek yogurt or a small scoop of frozen yogurt.

1 large pineapple, core removed, cut into rings
Ground cinnamon

1. Heat a grill pan over medium heat. Grill the pineapple rings for 2 to 3 minutes per side.

2. While still warm, sprinkle with cinnamon.

PER SERVING (WITHOUT YOGURT): Calories: 105; Total Fat: 0g; Saturated Fat: 0g; Carbohydrates: 27g; Fiber: 0g; Protein: 1g

BAKED APPLES

SERVES 4; PREP TIME: 5 MINUTES
COOK TIME: 30 MINUTES

A stellar alternative to apple pie, these baked apples are steamed in apple cider, which warm the cinnamon. If you like a little crunch, sprinkle with chopped walnuts after baking.

2 apples, cut in half crosswise

2 tablespoon butter or coconut oil

½ cup apple cider or water

Ground cinnamon

1. Preheat the oven to 350°F.

2. Place the apples cut-side up in a baking dish.

3. Top each apple half with a pat of butter. Pour the apple cider into the baking dish. Sprinkle with cinnamon. Cover with aluminum foil.

4. Bake for 30 to 35 minutes or until the apples are tender and bubbly.

TIP: This recipe also works with pears. You may need to adjust the cooking time since pears tend to cook faster.

PER SERVING: Calories: 113; Total Fat: 6g; Saturated Fat: 4g; Carbohydrates: 15g; Fiber: 2g; Protein: 0g

CHOCOLATE CHIA PUDDING

SERVES 4; PREP TIME: 5 MINUTES,
PLUS 4 HOURS CHILLING TIME
COOK TIME: NONE

Nutrient-rich chia seeds absorb liquid and swell up, creating a custard without using any eggs. This recipe creates a chocolate pudding that's packed with important nutrients like omega-3 fats and fiber to help support healthy circulation and digestion.

3 cups chocolate soy milk

¾ cup chia seeds

¼ cup sliced almonds

1. In a large bowl, combine the soy milk and chia seeds. Mix well to combine.

2. Pour mixture into four small bowls. Transfer to the refrigerator and allow to set for 2 hours.

3. After 2 hours, stir the contents of each bowl and allow to chill for 2 more hours.

4. Top with sliced almonds before serving.

PER SERVING: Calories: 224; Total Fat: 10g; Saturated Fat: 0g; Carbohydrates: 30g; Fiber: 11g; Protein: 10g

ZUCCHINI BREAD

MAKES 1 LOAF (12 SLICES);
PREP TIME: 15 MINUTES
COOK TIME: 45 MINUTES

Every family kitchen needs a zucchini bread recipe for those warm summer months when the garden is bursting with summer squash. This bread can also serve as breakfast when accompanied by fruit and yogurt. To make it a bit sweeter for dessert, toss some mini chocolate chips into the batter before baking.

Olive oil, for the loaf pan

2 cups whole-wheat pastry flour

¾ teaspoon ground cinnamon

½ teaspoon baking soda

¼ teaspoon kosher salt

½ cup pure maple syrup

4 tablespoons coconut oil

½ cup applesauce

1 teaspoon pure vanilla extract

1¼ cups grated zucchini

1. Preheat the oven to 350°F. Grease the inside of a loaf pan with a small amount of olive oil and set aside.

2. In a large bowl, whisk together the flour, cinnamon, baking soda, and salt, and set aside.

3. Using an electric mixer and a mixing bowl, combine the maple syrup and coconut oil. Add the applesauce and vanilla, and mix on low speed until well combined.

4. Slowly add the flour mixture into the applesauce mixture and mix until just combined. Fold in the zucchini.

5. Transfer the batter to the prepared pan. Bake until the batter mounds up and a cake tester comes out clean, about 45 minutes.

6. Cool in the pan for 15 minutes. Remove from the pan and transfer to a cooling rack to cool completely.

PER SLICE: Calories: 157; Total Fat: 5g; Saturated Fat: 4g; Carbohydrates: 26g; Fiber: 2g; Protein: 3g

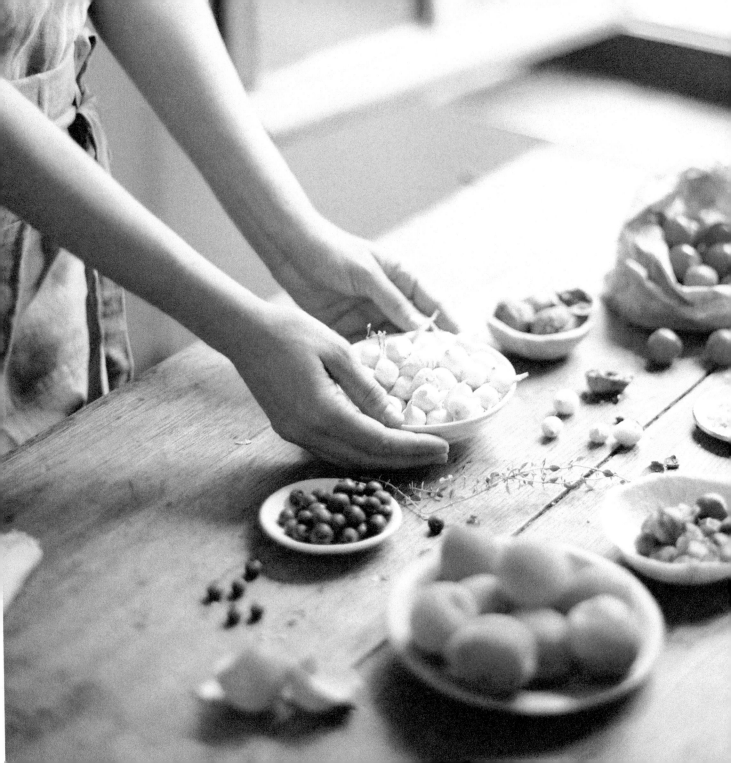

References

Academy of Breastfeeding Medicine Protocol Committee. "Clinical Protocol #9: Use of Galactogogues in Initiating or Augmenting the Rate of Maternal Milk Secretion." *Breastfeeding Medicine* 6 (2011): 41–9.

Allen, S. J., S. Jordan, M. Storey, C. A. Thornton, M. Gravenor, I. Garaiova, et al. "Dietary Supplementation with Lactobacilli and Bifidobacteria Is Well Tolerated and Not Associated with Adverse Events During Late Pregnancy and Early Infancy." *Journal of Nutrition* 140 (2010): 483–8.

American Congress of Obstetrics and Gynecology. "Committee Opinion No 267: Exercise During Pregnancy and the Postpartum Period." ACOG *Obstetrics and Gynecology* 99 (2002): 171–3.

American Congress of Obstetrics and Gynecology. "Committee Opinion Number 548: Weight Gain During Pregnancy." January 2013.

American Congress of Obstetrics and Gynecology. "Committee Opinion Number 549: Obesity in Pregnancy." *Obstetrics and Gynecology* 121, no. 1 (2013): 213–17.

American Congress of Obstetrics and Gynecology. "Practice Bulletin Number 52: Nausea and Vomiting of Pregnancy." *Obstetrics and Gynecology* 103 (2004): 803–13.

Aris, A., and S. Leblanc. "Maternal and Fetal Exposure to Pesticides Associated with Genetically Modified Foods in Eastern Townships of Quebec, Canada." *Reproductive Toxicology* 31, no. 4 (May 2011): 528–33.

Berggren, A., A. I. Lazou, N. Larsson, et al. "Randomized, Double-Blind and Placebo-Controlled Study Using New Probiotic Lactobacilli for Strengthening the Body Immune Defense against Viral Infections." *European Journal of Nutrition* 50 (2011): 203–10.

Bleich, S. N., W. L. Bennett, K. A. Gudzune, and L. A. Cooper. "Impact of Physician BMI on Obesity Care and Beliefs." *Obesity* 20, no. 5 (May 2012): 999–1005.

Booney, C. M., A. Verma, R. Tucker, et al. "Metabolic Syndrome in Childhood: Association with Birth Weight, Maternal Obesity, and Gestational Diabetes Mellitus." *Pediatrics* 115, no. 3 (2005): 290–6.

Castiglioni, S., A. Cazzaniga, W. Albisetti, et al. "Magnesium and Osteoporosis: Current State of Knowledge and Future Research Directions." *Nutrients* 5, no. 8 (August 2013): 3022–33.

Coyle, C. W., K. E. Wisner, K. L. Driscoll, and C. T. Clark. "Placentophagy: Therapeutic Miracle or Myth?" *Archives of Women's Mental Health* 18, no. 5 (October 2015): 673–80.

Craig, W. J., and A. R. Mangels. "Position of the American Dietetic Association: Vegetarian Diets." *Journal of the American Dietetic Association* 109, no. 7 (July 2009): 1266–82.

Crinnion, W. J. "Organic Foods Contain Higher Levels of Certain Nutrients, Lower Levels of Pesticides, and May Provide Health Benefits for the Consumer." *Alternate Medicine Review* 15, no. 1 (April 2010): 4–12.

De-Regil, L., C. Palacios, L.K. Lombardo, J. Pena-Rosas. "Vitamin D Supplementation for Women During Pregnancy." *Cochrane Database Systematic Reviews* 2 (2016).

Dinatale A., S. Ermito, I. Fonti, et al. "Obesity and Fetal-Maternal Outcomes." *Journal of Perinatal Medicine* 4, no. 1 (Jan–Mar 2010): 5–8.

Ding, X. X., Y. L. Wu, S. J. Xu, R. P. Zhu, et al. "Maternal Anxiety During Pregnancy and Adverse Birth Outcomes: A Systematic Review and Meta-Analysis of Prospective Cohort Studies." *Journal of Affect Disord* 159 (April 2014): 103–10.

Fasano, A., A. Sapone, V. Zevallos, and D. Schuppan. "Nonceliac Gluten Sensitivity." *Gastroenterology* 148, no. 6 (May 2015): 1195–204.

Fisher, N., P. Lattimore, and P. Malinowski. "Attention with a Mindful Attitude Attenuates Subjective Appetitive Reactions and Food Intake Following Food-Cue Exposure." *Appetite* 1, no. 99 (April 2016): 10–16.

Flaxman, S. M., and P. W. Sherman. "Morning Sickness: Adaptive Cause or Nonadaptive Consequence of Embryo Viability?" *The American Naturalist* 172, no. 1 (July 2008): 54–62.

Fyfe, E. M., J. M. Thompson, N. H. Anderson, et al. "Maternal Obesity and Postpartum Haemorrhage After Vaginal and Caesarean Delivery Among Nulliparous Women at Term: A Retrospective Cohort Study." *BMC Pregnancy and Childbirth* 12 (2012): 112.

Gearhardt, A. N., W. R. Corbin, and K. D. Brownell. "Preliminary Validation of the Yale Food Addiction Scale." *Appetite* 52, no. 2 (April 2009): 430–36.

Georgieff, Michael K. "Nutrition and the Developing Brain: Nutrient Priorities and Measurement." *American Journal of Clinical Nutrition* 85 (2007; supplement): 614S–20S.

Gibson, K. S., T. P. Waters, D. D. Gunzler, and P. M. Catalano. "A Retrospective Cohort Study of Factors Relating to the Longitudinal Change in Birth Weight." *BMC Pregnancy Childbirth* 15 (2015): 344.

Gupta, R. K., S. Singh, S. Gangoliya, and N. K. Singh. "Reduction of Phytic Acid and Enhancement of Bioavailable Micronutrients in Food Grains." *Journal of Food Science and Technology* 52, no. 2 (February 2015): 676–84.

Hardy, M. L. "Women's Health Series: Herbs of Special Interest to Women." *Journal of the American Pharmacology Association* 40 (2000): 234–42.

Hausner, H., W. L. Bredie, C. Molgaard, et al. "Differential Transfer of Dietary Flavour Compounds into Human Breast Milk." *Physiological Behavior* 95 (2009): 118–24.

Heringhausen, J. and K.S. Montgomery. "Continuing Education Module—Maternal Calcium Intake and Metabolism During Pregnancy and Lactation." *Journal of Perinatal Education* 14, no. 1 (Winter 2005): 52–57.

Howie, G., D. M. Sloboda, T. Kamal, and M. H. Vickers. "Maternal Nutritional History Predicts Obesity in Adult Offspring Independent of Postnatal Diet." *Journal of Physiology* 587, no. 4 (2009): 905–15.

Jayaprakasam, B., L. K. Olson, R. E. Schutzki, M. H. Tai, and M. G. Nair. "Amelioration of Obesity and Glucose Intolerance in High Fat Fed C57BL/6 Mice by Anthocyanins and Ursolic Acid in Cornelian Cherry (Cornus mas)." *Journal of Agricultural Food Chemistry*, 54 (2006): 243–48.

Jiang, C. B., C. Y. Yeh, H. C. Lee, et al. "Mercury Concentration in Meconium and Risk Assessment of Fish Consumption Among Pregnant Women in Taiwan." *Science of Total Environment* 408, no. 3 (January 2010): 518–23.

Johnson, R. K., L. J. Appel, M. Brands, et al. "Dietary Sugars Intake and Cardiovascular Health: A Scientific Statement from the American Heart Association." *Circulation* 120, no. 11 (September 15, 2009): 1011–20.

Johnston, B. C., A. L. Supina, M. Ospina, S. Vohra. "Probiotics for the Prevention of Pediatric Antibiotic-Associated Diarrhea." Cochrane Database Syst Rev. 2 (April 18, 2007): CD004827.

Kafaei Atrian, M., Z. Sadat, M. Rasolzadeh Bidgoly, F. Abbaszadeh, and M. Asghari Jafarabadi. "The Association of Sexual Intercourse During Pregnancy with Labor Onset." *Iran Red Crescent Medical Journal* 17, no. 1 (December 26, 2014): e16465.

Koufman, J. A. "Low-Acid Diet for Recalcitrant Laryngopharyngeal Reflux: Therapeutic Benefits and Their Implications." *Annals of Otology, Rhinology & Laryngology* 120, no. 5 (May 2011): 281–87.

Lam, J., L. Kelly, C. Ciszkowski, et al. "Central Nervous System Depression of Neonates Breastfed by Mothers Receiving Oxycodone for Postpartum Analgesia." *Journal of Pediatrics* 160 (2012): 33–37.

Lassi, Z. S., A. M. Imam, S. V. Dean, and Z. A. Bhutta. "Preconception Care: Caffeine, Smoking, Alcohol, Drugs and Other Environmental Chemical/Radiation Exposure." *Reproductive Health* 11, Supplement 3 (2014): 6.

Laugeray, A., A. Herzine, O. Perche, et al. "Pre- and Postnatal Exposure to Low Dose Glufosinate Ammonium Induces Autism-Like Phenotypes in Mice." *Frontiers in Behavioral Neuroscience* 20, no. 8 (November 2014): 390.

Lee Y. M, S. A. Kim, I. K. Lee, et al. "Effect of a Brown Rice Based Vegan Diet and Conventional Diabetic Diet on Glycemic Control of Patients with Type 2 Diabetes: A 12-Week Randomized Clinical Trial." *PLOS One* 11 (2016): e0155918.

Liu, S., R. M. Liston, K. S. Joseph, M. Heaman, R. Sauve, R., and M. S. Kramer. "Maternal Mortality and Severe Morbidity Associated with Low-Risk Planned Cesarean Delivery Versus Planned Vaginal Delivery at Term." *Canadian Medical Association Journal* 176, no. 4 (2007): 455–60.

Maruyama, K., T. Oshima, and K. Ohyama. "Exposure to Exogenous Estrogen Through Intake of Commercial Milk Produced from Pregnant Cows." *Pediatrics International* 52, no. 1, (February 2010): 33–38.

Matthews, A., D. M. Haas, D. P. O'Mathuna, et al. "Interventions for Nausea and Vomiting in Early Pregnancy." *The Cochrane Database of Systematic Reviews* 3 (2014): CD007575.

Mennella, J. A., M. S. Jagnow, and G. K. Beauchamp. "Prenatal and Postnatal Flavor Learning by Human Infants." *Pediatrics* 107, no. 6 (June 2001): E88.

Moore, Keith L., ed. *The Developing Human: Clinically Oriented Embryology*. 9th ed. Amsterdam: Elsevier, 2013.

Nettleton, J. A., P. L. Lutsey, Y. Wang, et al. "Diet Soda Intake and Risk of Incident Metabolic Syndrome and Type 2 Diabetes in the Multi-Ethnic Study of Atherosclerosis (MESA)." *Diabetes Care* 32, no. 4 (April 2009): 688–94.

Niazi, A. K., and S. K. Niazi. "Mindfulness-Based Stress Reduction: A Non-Pharmacological Approach for Chronic Illnesses." *North American Journal of Medical Science* 3, no. 1 (January 2011): 20–3.

Noren, K. "Levels of Organochlorine Contaminants in Human Milk in Relation to the Dietary Habits of the Mothers." *Acta Paediatrica Scandinavia* 72, no. 6 (November 1983): 811–6.

O'Connor, P. J., and T. W. Puetz. "Chronic Physical Activity and Feelings of Energy and Fatigue." *Medical Science Sports Exercise* 37, no. 2 (2005): 299–305.

Piccoli, G. B., R. Clari, F. N. Vigotti, et al. "Vegan-Vegetarian Diets in Pregnancy: Danger or Panacea?" *BJOG* 122, no. 5 (April 2015): 623–33.

Ramirez, G. B., M. C. Cruz, O. Pagulayan, E. Ostrea, and C. Dalisay. "The Tagum Study I: Analysis and Clinical Correlates of Mercury in Maternal and Cord Blood, Breast Milk, Meconium, and Infants' Hair." *Pediatrics* 106, no. 4 (October 2000): 774–81.

Ramirez, G. B., O. Pagulayan, H. Akagi, et al. "Tagum Study II: Follow-Up Study at Two Years of Age After Prenatal Exposure to Mercury." *Pediatrics* 111, no. 3 (March 2003): 289–95.

Rasmussen, K. M., and A. L. Yaktine, editors. *Weight Gain During Pregnancy: Reexamining the Guidelines.* Washington, DC: National Academies Press, 2009.

Reynolds, C. M., M. H. Vickers, C. J. Harrison, S. A. Segovia, and C. Gray. "High Fat and/or High Salt Intake During Pregnancy Alters Maternal Meta-Inflammation and Offspring Growth and Metabolic Profiles." *Physiological Reports* 2, no. 8 (August 2014).

Sachs, H. C. "The Transfer of Drugs and Therapeutics into Human Breast Milk: An Update on Selected Topics." *Pediatrics* 132 (2013): 796–809.

Samsel, A, and S. Seneff. "Glyphosate, Pathways to Modern Diseases II: Celiac Sprue and Gluten Intolerance." *Interdisciplinary Toxicology* 6, no. 4 (December 2013): 159–84.

Sayers, A., and J. H. Tobias. "Estimated Maternal Ultraviolet B Exposure Levels in Pregnancy Influence Skeletal Development of the Child." *Journal of Clinical Endocrinoloy & Metabolism* 94, no. 3 (March 2009): 765–71.

Schaffir, J. "Sexual Intercourse at Term and Onset of Labor." *Obstetrics & Gynecology* 107 (2006): 1310.

Seaton, S., M. Reeves, and S. McLean. "Oxycodone as a Component of Multimodal Analgesia for Lactating Mothers after Caesarean Section: Relationships between Maternal Plasma, Breast Milk and Neonatal Plasma Levels." *Australia & New Zealand Journal of Obstetrics & Gynaecology* 47 (2007): 181–85.

Sherman, P. W., and S. M. Flaxman. "Nausea and Vomiting of Pregnancy in An Evolutionary Perspective." *American Journal of Obstetrics & Gynecology* 186, no. 5 (May 2002): 190–97.

Smith-Spangler, C., M. L. Brandeau, G. E. Hunter, et al. "Are Organic Foods Safer or Healthier Than Conventional Alternatives? A Systematic Review." *Annals of Internal Medicine* 157, no. 5 (September 4, 2012): 348–66.

Springmann, M., H. C. J. Godfray, M. Rayner, and P. Scarborough. "Analysis and Valuation of the Health and Climate Change Cobenefits of Dietary Change." *Proceedings of the National Academy of Sciences* 113, no. 15 (April 2016): 4146–51.

Staples, J., A. Ponsonby, and L. Lim. "Low Maternal Exposure to Ultraviolet Radiation in Pregnancy, Month of Birth, and Risk of Multiple Sclerosis in Offspring: Longitudinal Analysis." *BMJ* 340 (2010): c1640.

Thomson, M., R. Corbin, and L. Leung. "Effects of Ginger for Nausea and Vomiting in Early Pregnancy: A Meta-Analysis." *Journal of the American Board of Family Medicine* 27, no. 1 (2014): 115–22.

Tuso, P. J., M. H. Ismail, B. P. Ha, and C. Bartolotto. "Nutritional Update for Physicians: Plant-Based Diets." *Permanente Journal* 17, no. 2 (Spring 2013): 61–66

Young, S. M., and D. C. Benyshek. "In Search of Human Placentophagy: A Cross-Cultural Survey of Human Placenta Consumption, Disposal Practices, and Cultural Beliefs." *Ecology of Food and Nutrition* 49, no. 6 (November-December 2010): 467–84.

Resources

AMERICAN CONGRESS
OF OBSTETRICIANS AND
GYNECOLOGISTS
acog.org/patients

BMI CALCULATOR
webmd.com/diet/
body-bmi-calculator

DIETARY REFERENCE
INTAKE TABLES
nationalacademies.org/
hmd/activities/nutrition/
summaryDRIs/DRI-Tables

ENVIRONMENTAL
WORKING GROUP
ewg.org

FERMENTING
paleoleap.com/
fermented-food-recipes/

THE INSTITUTE FOR
RESPONSIBLE NUTRITION
responsiblefoods.org

LOCAL GROWERS,
MARKETPLACES, AND EVENTS
localharvest.com

ORGANIC PASTURED MEATS
eatwild.com

PHYSICIANS COMMITTEE FOR
RESPONSIBLE MEDICINE
pcrm.org

THE PUMP STATION
(Breast-feeding and new
mother resource)
pumpstation.com

SPROUTING FOODS
sproutpeople.org

THRIVE MARKET
(Non-produce organic
items with free shipping)
thrivemarket.com

VEGAN BAKING
veganbaking.net

VEGAN HEALTH
veganhealth.org

THE VEGETARIAN
RESOURCE GROUP
vrg.org

THE WORLD'S
HEALTHIEST FOODS
whfoods.org

YOFFIE LIFE
(Wellness site including
nutrition, recipes, and
other subjects)
yoffielife.com

Recipe Index

Index

Acknowledgments

There are so many people who are lights in my life and without whom I could not have pulled this off.

Foremost I would like to acknowledge Dana White, a phenomenal chef and food educator. Without her aesthetically beautiful, nutrition-packed menu this book would be rather bland. She shows us all how healthy eating can be fun, easy, and delicious.

I owe an enormous debt of gratitude to my friend Pamela Kawada, who (after years of listening to my diatribes about healthy eating) encouraged me to put my passion on paper and helped set this entire process in motion.

Thanks to my incredible editor, Meg Ilasco, and the entire team at Callisto Media. Your visionary approach to publishing is disrupting the industry for good reason. Thanks for believing in this project, and in me.

I am so grateful to all the revolutionaries out there working every day to counter the wave of misinformation coming from big agribusiness and the food industry. You are my heroes and my inspiration. We do not have to accept the status quo of rising obesity, diabetes, and other diet-related illness, including cancer. Our children deserve better.

Gratitude to my many friends in the birthing community, most especially to Dr. Eliot Berlin, Dr. Stuart Fischbein, Deborah Frank, Dr. Michelle Gerber, Alisha Tamburri, Ricki Lake, and Dr. Jennifer Margulis. You are all passionate advocates for women's empowerment and informed consent, which begins with knowing what we are putting into our bodies on a daily basis through our foods. I acknowledge and hold sacred all the deep wisdom passed down through the centuries by midwives and doulas. It's exciting to watch the science slowly catch up.

Special thanks to my friends at The Honest Company, especially the incredible authors and entrepreneurs Christopher Gavigan and Jessica Alba. Your books inspired me to write this, and your products make it a little easier for all of us to be good to our bodies, our babies, and the planet.

Thank you to all my fellow mom-activists. Your companies, films and TV shows, nonprofits, books, law practices, medical practices, and lives are a constant source of battery charge for me. With all this love for our children and the planet, righteous indignation, and countless graduate degrees amongst us, I'm pretty sure we're actually going to change the world.

And finally, thanks to my amazing husband, Peter, and miraculous kids Sheila, Nico, and Sofia. You guys are my everything. Love All Around.

CPSIA information can be obtained
at www.ICGtesting.com
Printed in the USA
BVOW10s1742110417
480839BV00001B/1/P